Menopause
and
Estrogen

Menopause and Estrogen

Natural Alternatives to Hormome Replacement Therapy

Ellen H. Brown

and

Lynne P. Walker, Pharm.D., M.Ac., D.H.M.

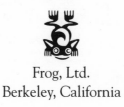

Frog, Ltd.
Berkeley, California

Notice to the Reader

This book is not intended to replace good medical diagnosis and treatment. Its purpose is to help you work with your health care practitioner in making informed treatment decisions.

Menopause and Estrogen: Natural Alternatives to Hormone Replacement Therapy

Copyright © 1996 by Ellen Hodgson Brown. No portion of this book, except for brief review, may be reproduced, stored in a retrieval system, or transmitted, in any form or by any means, electronic, mechanical, photocopying, recording or otherwise without the written permission of the publisher. For information contact Frog, Ltd. c/o North Atlantic Books.

Published by
Frog, Ltd.

Frog, Ltd. Books are distributed by
North Atlantic Books
P.O. Box 12327
Berkeley, California 94712

Cover and book design by Paula Morrison
Typeset by Catherine Campaigne
Printed in the United States of America

Distributed to the book trade by Publisher's Group West

Library of Congress Cataloging-in-Publication Data

Brown, Ellen Hodgson.
    Menopause and estrogen : natural alternatives to hormone replacement
therapy / Ellen H. Brown and Lynne P. Walker. — 2nd rev. ed.
        p.   cm.
    Formerly published in 1994 under the title : Breezing through the change :
managing menopause naturally.
    Includes bibliographical references and index.
    ISBN 1-883319-53-6
    1. Menopause—Complications—Alternative treatment.   2. Premenstrual
syndrome—Alternative treatment.   I. Walker, Lynne Paige.   II. Brown, Ellen
Hodgson.   Breezing through the change.   III. Title.
RG186.B76   1997
618.1'75—dc21   96-53863
                                                                                        CIP

            3   4   5   6   7   8   9   10 / 04   03   02   01   00

Table of Contents

Charts and Diagrams

Foreword

Everyday is a surprise, more so with each passing year. There is so much more to remember and to learn. New windows are opening into understanding women's life-changes, physically, psychically, and societally. Enjoy your journey, the path is rich and deep.

My medical training prepared me poorly with respect to many women's health care issues, especially menopause. It seemed cut and dried: "Ovarian failure." "Dried up." All downhill from there. Thank goodness they were wrong.

Menopause, as I have come to learn, marks a time in life of shifting strengths and purposes, from earth mother to wise woman. When I look around at my friends and myself, I see a lot more that is deepening than our wrinkles. "Second spring" is a term that suits me.

The medical approach to menopause involves an archaic conception of female endocrinology as purely chemical. Today many educated women are searching for choices more compatible with our nature. More than one million women are now turning fifty each year. They include doctors, lawyers, and corporate executives. We now have an opportunity to reevaluate this natural transition with new eyes and more sophisticated testing. At the same time, the long-ignored healing powers of the plant kingdom are rapidly coming back into popular knowledge and use.

Competing with this natural approach, the drug companies involved in marketing synthetic hormonal products are investing massive amounts of money in proving that their products are the *only* choice a woman has, and in downplaying their products' dangers. They are creating a standard of care among physicians and falsely frightening women into complying: ERT (Estrogen Replacement Therapy) or dry up and die prematurely.

Menopause and Estrogen (formerly *Breezing Through the Change*) starts out by dispelling that myth. It transcends the dark ages of menopause, returning to women their rightful power to care for themselves. The book advises women on what their best options are today, supported by the latest research. These alternatives include herbal and homeopathic products, natural hormones derived from plants, and healthy lifestyle options.

As a physician who advises in the use of natural methods and remedies whenever they are appropriate as an option, I heartily welcome this outstanding book. I have longed for *one book* that would explain and document the myriad choices we have and their inherent risk or lack of risk. For patients and practitioners alike, this book is educational and practical. I will use it as a handbook for all women interested "in the Change."

We now know that the end of menses is not the beginning of menopause but merely a point in the passage. Disturbed sleep, night sweats, irregular periods, and emotional changes often precede the last period; while hormone levels start changing as early as our thirties, producing the symptoms we call PMS. These changes are significant and need attention for our long-term best interest. Many cultures, including the Chinese, respect and understand these more subtle changes and have created tonics for them. American Indian women knew the hormonal properties of their local plants and how to use them. In most cultures, it has been women who knew which herbs to use for healing and educated one another from generation to generation. It is fitting that we take this knowledge once again into our own hands.

—Jesse Hanley, M.D.
Malibu, California

Introduction to the Second Edition

In the two years since this book first was published, we have become even more excited about the natural remedies it discusses. In my own case, apparently due to the consistent use of a natural progesterone skin cream, a large fibroid tumor that my gynecologist said would "have to come out" has "spontaneously" vanished; I have succeeded in avoiding a recommended hysterectomy for uterine prolapse; and I have thrown away a wrist brace that I had worn every night for seventeen years for carpal tunnel syndrome.

Dr. Walker has seen many more such remarkable results in her practice as a homeopath and as proprietress of Sun Valley Herb Company in Sun Valley, Idaho. She has observed about thirty cases in which carpal tunnel syndrome was reversed using natural progesterone alone. This dramatic effect does not seem to have been previously reported. In a typical case, a 68-year-old woman was concerned that she was about to lose her job at a local grocery store because she could not lift products onto the shelves. Dr. Walker recommended that the woman rub ¼ teaspoon of natural progesterone cream on her wrist twice a day until asymptomatic, then use that amount once a day (not necessarily on the hands). In 3½ weeks, the woman's carpal tunnel problem had resolved and her job was secure.

Other notable results observed by Dr. Walker include the elimination of vaginal dryness with the use of Ostaderm V vaginal plant estrogen/progesterone cream; the reversal of insomnia and dry skin with the oral use of evening primrose oil; and the disappearance of arthritic symptoms with the application of natural progesterone cream directly to the affected site.

Note, however, that not all products that claim to contain progesterone seem to be effective. Some contain ingredients that may be toxic. Two products we have found to be effective are Pro-Gest, distributed by Transitions for Health, and one called simply Yam Cream, distributed by Pacific Research Laboratories (see Appendix). Studies on hormone research in the last two years report both good and bad news. New studies have solidified the link between breast cancer and conventional estrogen. However, the natural plant estrogens and progesterones don't seem to be linked to cancer and may afford protection against it.

Estrogen and breast cancer

The ongoing Nurses' Health Study, involving 121,700 women, has been given considerable credence because of its size and location in the United States. Its latest findings, reported in June of 1995, were that women who took estrogen after menopause had a 32 percent higher risk of breast cancer than those who hadn't taken the hormone. Women aged 50 to 64 who had used hormones for 5 to 9 years had a 46 percent increased risk, and women aged 60 to 64 using hormones for five years or more had a 71 percent increased risk. The study also found a 45 percent increased risk of death from breast cancer in women who had taken estrogen for five years or longer. Women who had been off the drugs for two years or more, however, showed no increased risk.

The bottom line seems to be that taking estrogen for a few years to relieve hot flashes and other acute symptoms of menopause is safe; but taking it for decades, e.g. to ward off osteoporosis and heart disease, may be asking for trouble. The problem is that to slow bone loss, estrogen *must* be taken for decades. In women who stop taking it after menopause, bone loss resumes and eventually catches up to the level of women who have never taken it.[1]

The Nurses' Health Study also dashed hopes that taking synthetic progestins with estrogen (the combination called HRT) would counteract estrogen's effects in stimulating tumors in the breast, as it does for tumors in the uterus. Women on HRT actually had a *greater* risk of developing breast cancer than women on estrogen alone.[2]

Increased estrogen use, of course, isn't the only suspect in the precipitous rise in breast cancer rates. Other causes lately in the news include high-fat diets; DDT and other environmental toxins, which act as "pseudoestrogens" that accumulate in the fat cells of the breast; and mass screening, which has inflated the figures with false positive findings and pre-cancerous lumps that might never have gone on to become serious disease. The increased risk of breast cancer for women on estrogen is still a significant one, which has to be weighed against the hormone's touted but not-yet-proven benefits.

Estrogen and heart disease

On the benefits side, on January 18, 1995, *JAMA* reported the results of the Postmenopausal Estrogen/Progestin Interventions (PEPI) Trial, the first randomized, double-blind, placebo-controlled prospective study of the effects of estrogen on cholesterol and triglyceride levels. It found that estrogen significantly increased levels of high-density lipoprotein cholesterol (HDL-C, the "good" cholesterol). HDL-C is thought to be the best predictor of heart disease risk in women: the higher the HDL-C, the lower the risk.

Confounding the issue, however, was the fact that triglycerides also went up in women on estrogen, suggesting an *increase* in heart disease risk. And taking synthetic progestins with the estrogen—the HRT protocol popular in the United States—reduced the HDL-C benefit of estrogen used alone by a full 75 percent.

A second PEPI report, issued in the *Journal of the American Medical Association (JAMA)* on February 7, 1996, strongly advised women with intact uteruses not to take estrogen alone. The report looked at studies of endometrial hyperplasia, a condition involving excessive growth of the uterine lining which is considered to be a precursor of uterine cancer. The studies compared the uterine linings of women on (a) a placebo, (b) estrogen alone, (c) an estrogen/progestin combination, and (d) an estrogen/natural progesterone combination. Only 2 of 119 women on the placebo developed endometrial hyperplasia, and no more than 6 women developed it in the estrogen/progesterone groups. But *seventy-four* women—or nearly two-thirds—developed the condition on estrogen alone.

Women sometimes choose to take estrogen alone because they can't stand the side effects of synthetic progestins, but these side effects can be avoided by using natural progesterone. Until recently, the effectiveness of natural progesterone in staving off uterine cancer hadn't been proven; but in this second PEPI report, natural progesterone was indeed found to be as effective as synthetic progestins for this purpose.[3]

Other positive findings involving natural progesterone came from the first PEPI report. While *synthetic* progestins reduced estrogen's benefits on HDL-C levels by 75 percent, *natural* progesterone did not have this effect.[4]

What remains to be proven is that estrogen actually reduces heart disease incidence. The Women's Health Initiative (WHI), the first widely approved controlled clinical trial designed to resolve these questions, won't issue even preliminary findings until 1999. Meanwhile, estrogen's dire effect on cancer rates has been established; and experts are predicting that cancer will have overtaken heart disease as the number one killer by the year 2000.[5] "Basically," observed Dr. Isaac Schiff, chief of obstetrics and gynecology at Massachusetts General Hospital, "you're presenting women with the possibility of increasing the risk of getting breast cancer at age 60 in order to prevent a heart attack at age 70 and a hip fracture at age 80."[6]

Estrogen versus progesterone in the battle against osteoporosis

Estrogen is currently being prescribed long-term to ward off not only heart disease but osteoporosis. Estimated U.S. sales of estrogen and other osteoporosis drugs topped a billion dollars in 1994 and are predicted to reach $3.3 billion before the year 2000. One reason for estrogen's popularity is the dearth of viable alternatives. Until recently, it was the only drug that was FDA-approved for treating osteoporosis. However, two other drugs have now been approved: alendronate (Fosamex), a nonhormonal product; and a salmon calcitonin nasal spray (Miacalcin).

A major drawback of these newer options is their price: they are more than five times as expensive as Premarin, which already costs up to $30 per month.[7] A cheaper alternative that is not accompanied by either side effects or the risk of breast cancer is discussed in Chapter 9. In a study conducted by John Lee, M.D., natural progesterone was shown to have an even more favorable effect than estrogen on bone density. A new Dutch study reported in 1994 augmented this research, finding that progesterone actually outperforms estrogen in stimulating the proliferation of the cells that form new bone.[8]

So why has natural progesterone been overlooked by the media? Probably because it is outside the major pharmaceutical loop and therefore little known. Manufacturers of natural remedies, which lack the massive funding required for FDA approval, were until recently prohibited by FDA regulations from making claims about their products. Those rules changed with the Dietary Supplement Health Act of 1994, which allowed natural supplements to bear claims that were truthful and not misleading. Manufacturers have been slow to capitalize on this change in the law, mainly because of uncertainty about how it will be interpreted. The FDA can still ban supplements via several loopholes, including controversial safety issues based on anonymous toxicity reports; and state regulations may still apply. There is also the concern that the FDA might consider even medical research "misleading," if it disagrees with prior research and conventional wisdom.[9]

Natural progesterone, however, may soon be in the major media loop. Wyeth-Ayerst (maker of Premarin) has invested $9.5 million in developing Crinone, a sustained-release, vaginal natural progesterone product that has a patented "bioadhesive" delivery system. Crinone has already been approved in France, the U.K. and Finland for various indications, including the prevention of hyperplasia and endometrial cancer in women on HRT, the treatment of PMS, dysfunctional uterine bleeding, and infertility due to inadequate progesterone production.[10]

Estrogen and Alzheimer's

A third long-term indication for estrogen has been lately in the news: it may help ward off Alzheimer's disease. In an ongoing study of female residents at a California retirement community called Leisure World, investigators compared 127 Leisure World decedents whose death certificates mentioned Alzheimer's or dementia with the matched records of decedents who hadn't died of either cause. They found that estrogen users were 40 percent less likely than non-users to have died of either condition. The researchers also found that Alzheimer's patients on estrogen performed better on a standard mental exam than patients who weren't on estrogen.

Alas, it is the nature of empirical science that for every study that goes one way, another is liable to go the other way. In a quite similar study involving residents of Rancho San Bernardo, California, women decedents who had been taking estrogen were found to be almost twice as likely to have died of Alzheimer's disease as women who hadn't taken it! Further, when the researchers compared the test scores for memory and mental acuity of women on estrogen and women not on it, no significant differences were found.[11]

Neither study was a controlled clinical trial (in which two groups of postmenopausal women with similar baseline risks are randomly selected to receive either estrogen or a placebo). Patricia Fripp, writing in the *Harvard Women's Health Watch*, concludes, "Until there is information from the WHI [Women's Health Initiative] and other subsequent studies, Alzheimer's risk shouldn't weigh heavily in any woman's decision about hormone replacement therapy."[12]

Protection through diagnostic screening?

"[I]f I know hormones are going to protect my heart, my mind, and my bones," suggested Gail Sheehy in her book *The Silent Passage*, "I guess I can monitor my breasts with mammography and my uterus with ultrasound and see how it goes." However, as observed in a March 1994 article in *HealthFacts*:

> There's a downside to all screening programs: overdiagnosis and overtreatment... There are reports in the medical literature indicating that physician overreaction to microscopic lesions detected during Pap screening has caused many a woman to lose her uterus unnecessarily... It is possible that at least part of the rising cervical cancer incidence in young white women can be attributed to the misidentification of noninvasive lesions as cancer. This has clearly occurred in the nation's breast cancer statistics, which show a major increase in the rate of breast cancer that coincides with women's rising acceptance of mammography screening.[13]

False-positive readings can lead to unnecessary biopsies, invasive procedures that are not only painful but hazardous in themselves. There are three types of biopsies: excisional, incisional, and needle or aspiration biopsies. Excisional biopsies are considered the least likely to spread cancer, since they "excise" the whole tumor. But if the tumor is large, this is not a procedure you want to go through without first being sure the tumor is malignant. An alternative is incisional biopsy, in which only a chunk of the tumor is taken; but that means cutting right into the tumor. This is the very thing oncologists go to great lengths to avoid when doing cancer surgery, lest they spread the disease. The other alternative is needle biopsy, in which fluid or tissue is withdrawn through a needle for examination. That option is divided into fine needle and large needle biopsies, with the fine needle biopsy being considered the least likely to spread cancer. But studies have shown that all three biopsy options carry that risk.[14]

The controversy sparked by the National Breast Screening Study of Canada (NBSS) over whether women under fifty should receive routine mammography (discussed in Chapter 6) heated up dramatically in 1994. The National Cancer Institute, which launched the mammography crusade in the seventies, withdrew its long-standing endorsement that year of routine breast screening for these women, based on the conclusions of the 1993 International Workshop on Screening for Breast Cancer. The latter announced that for women aged 40–49, "randomized controlled trials of breast cancer screening showed no benefit 5–7 years after entry," while at 10–12 years, "benefit is uncertain and, if present marginal."[15] In an extensive exchange of correspondence reported in the *Journal of the National Cancer Institute* in November of 1994, NBSS head Dr. Anthony Miller observed that to justify mass screening, "[w]hat is necessary is demonstrated effectiveness in a population; regrettably, this evidence is not yet available for breast screening *for any age group*."[16]

In response, the National Women's Health Network and the Center for Medical Consumers began actively advising premenopausal women to *avoid* mammography, except to evaluate suspicious lumps. (They still recommend the procedure, however, for women over fifty.) Reasons younger women should think twice about mammography include:

1. It doesn't work well for them, since dense, healthy breast tissue can resemble or obscure tumors. In the Canadian study, routine mammography missed 40 percent of the breast cancers that developed in 25,000 women aged 40 to 49; and in a similar Swedish study, it missed 38 percent.

2. The Canadian study found that screening mammograms don't improve younger women's chances of survival.

3. Mammography exposes them to unnecessary radiation that may contribute to cancer growth. John Gofman, M.D., a University of California at Berkeley radiation researcher, has concluded that two-thirds of American breast cancer cases are due to x-rays received in the past.[17]

4. Mammography can result in false positive readings that lead to unnecessary biopsies.[18]

Vegetarian estrogen

Many women would rather suffer through their menopausal symptoms than risk breast cancer and the treatments for it that can be even more frightening than the disease. Choosing between these two options may no longer be necessary. For many women, natural progesterone alone will take care of their symptoms; and for women who need more, natural plant estrogens are now available. New research indicates that these plant estrogens, unlike animal and synthetic estrogens, not only aren't associated with increased rates of cancer of the breast and uterus but actually may afford protection against those diseases. Preliminary research also indicates that plant estrogens are as effective as, or more effective than, the conventional pharmaceutical options in increasing HDL (good cholesterol), lowering LDL (bad cholesterol), and causing arteries to constrict and dilate when they should.[19]

A review of study results published in the *Journal of Nutrition* in 1995 suggested that plant constituents called diphenolic isoflavonoids and lignans are converted by intestinal bacteria into hormone-like compounds with weak estrogenic activity. These compounds have been shown to influence sex hormone metabolism and to have biological effects that make them strong candidates as natural cancer fighters.[20] In premenopausal women, they seem to take the place of some of the body's own tumor-stimulating estrogen; while in postmenopausal women, they make up for the *lack* of the natural hormone, providing an estrogen lift without raising cancer risk.[21]

A study reported in the *New England Journal of Medicine* on

August 3, 1995 found that eating 47 grams of soy protein daily (about the amount in ¾ pound of firm tofu) also lowered cholesterol—by 20 percent in people whose levels were initially too high. In addition, soy protein significantly reduced LDL or "bad" cholesterol and triglycerides, both of which are primary heart disease risk factors. Again the effect was attributed to the phytoestrogen compounds called isoflavones. "These isoflavones," observed Dr. James Anderson, who helped conduct the study, "also may help reduce the risk of breast cancer and osteoporosis in women."[22]

Plant estrogens have the further advantage of being cruelty-free. Pregnant mare's urine, from which the leader among estrogens is derived, has become a huge commercial business that now caters to an estimated eight million women. The result has been to confine 75,000 mares to stalls hardly larger than themselves for months at a time, and to relegate tens of thousands of horses and foals annually to miserable lives and early deaths.[23]

So far, some 300 plants with estrogen-like activity have been identified, including carrots, corn, apples, barley, and oats. Soybean products like tofu seem to pack the strongest hormonal wallop; but not everyone likes tofu, and not all concentrated soy products contain the requisite isoflavones. If the soy protein in your soy burger, for example, has been extracted using alcohol rather than water, the isoflavones will largely have been lost.[24] Other problems with eating large amounts of soy are that soybeans grown in the U.S. are generally treated heavily with pesticides, and they can impair iron absorption, leading to anemia and iron deficiency in women.[25] Phytoestrogens absorbed through the skin in the form of transdermal creams, although not yet thoroughly tested, are an alternative that may avoid these problems (see Chapter 11).

Armed with the natural remedies discussed in this book, women no longer need fear "the Change." We can look forward to graduating from PMS to PMZ: what anthropologist Margaret Mead called "postmenopausal zest."

Introduction

No woman need suffer menopause or any of its symptoms if
she receives preventive treatment *before* the onset of menopause.... Every woman alive today has the option of remain-
ing feminine forever.
—Robert A. Wilson, M.D., 1966[1]

Unlike our grandmothers, who hesitated to discuss it, everyone is
now talking about menopause. Middle age has finally come to the
Baby Boomers. We were the Flower Power generation; we were never
going to get old. Now that we have, we're bent on finding innova-
tive ways to stall the inexorable march of time.

Motivated by the largest commercial market in history, the pharmaceutical industry has joined in the pursuit; and doctors have followed their lead. Forty million women are scheduled to go through
"the Change" in the next twenty years. Two or three million women
are already taking those patented hormones known as Estrogen
Replacement Therapy (ERT), and the drugs are typically prescribed
for life.

Yet a large market remains to be tapped, since these women represent only 15 percent of the potential market—down from 30 percent on ERT in the 1970s.[2]

To bridge the gap, estrogen is now being prescribed even for women
who breeze through menopause without symptoms, on the theory
that it will reduce their risks of heart disease and osteoporosis. Some
researchers, however, are uncomfortable with the assumptions. They
feel the benefits are uncertain, and the trade-off is an increased risk
of breast and uterine cancers.[3]

In the sixties, the chief proponent of ERT was Dr. Robert Wilson. In his trend-setting book *Feminine Forever*, he envisioned for
women a perennial youth maintained after menopause with supplemental estrogen. Dr. Wilson actually recommended that we start tak-

ing estrogen years *before* menopause—perhaps even in our thirties, when our hormone levels start to drop off—continuing into a youthful and sexy old age. But Dr. Wilson's vision faded in the face of the alarming increase in endometrial cancer (cancer of the lining of the uterus) that followed his recommendations. Although early reports of this risk surfaced in 1961, it wasn't until three studies strongly linking endometrial cancer to estrogen were reported in 1975 and 1976 that the Food and Drug Administration (FDA) recommended warnings on estrogen package inserts. Estrogen use then declined dramatically—by twenty-eight percent from 1975 to 1977.[4]

To temper that risk, after 1976 doctors routinely prescribed progestins along with estrogen. Progestins are synthetic forms of progesterone, the hormone that opposes the tumor-stimulating effects of estrogen in the body. But this too proved to be a solution with problems. The FDA has never approved the estrogen/progestin combination as hormone replacement therapy for postmenopausal women, so its long-term risks are unknown.[5] What research does show is that progestins may reverse the cardiovascular benefits of estrogen; and they do *not* reverse its increased risk of breast cancer and may increase it.[6] Synthetic progestins also come with a long list of side effects many women are unable or unwilling to endure.

Even with progestins, estrogen is no longer considered safe by most doctors until menstrual periods have entirely ceased. That means you may be denied this remedy not only as early as your thirties but when you're in the throes of "perimenopause" in your forties and fifties. Perimenopause is that time of life when your body is preparing for menopause but you're still having monthly periods. You may be experiencing some very distressing symptoms at that time, including hot flashes, vaginal dryness, loss of interest in sex, insomnia, and mood swings similar to premenstrual tension. But as estrogen researcher Lila Nachtigall, M.D., explains:

> This is no time to start estrogen replacement therapy even though you may desperately want it.... Today we know that, except under special circumstances, taking hormones before menopause, your very last menstrual period, can be dangerous. In fact, it can be especially dangerous during the erratic peri-

ods of perimenopause because that's a time when you may be producing huge amounts of estrogen in response to the frantic activities of the pituitary gland to get your ovaries back in business.[7]

The hard realities of estrogen's side effects and risks seem to have shattered forever the "feminine forever" ideal.

...Or have they? Could it be that Dr. Wilson was on the right track but had the wrong key? There *are* natural remedies that are safe and effective, not only after menopause but any time your hormones are out of balance. These natural remedies aren't widely publicized, but it's not because there isn't research in their favor. Their safety and effectiveness are supported by studies and clinical experience. They are not well known mainly because they are too inexpensive to interest the pharmaceutical companies that can afford to clear FDA hurdles. Since they are natural products, they can't be patented. Only synthetic substances—those *not* found naturally in plants or animals—can be patented, guaranteeing them a monopoly of the market. That means only patentable synthetics can generate sufficient profits to warrant investment in long-term studies. And without these studies (which in most cases must be privately funded), a remedy can't get FDA approval.

A popular misconception is that the FDA tests remedies, and if a remedy is safe and effective, the agency will find it and prove its worth. In fact, drug companies test their own remedies and submit the results to the FDA; and for a single drug, the average cost of these tests is now *over $100 million.*[8] That means small companies that cannot afford massive studies may have safe and effective remedies that do not have FDA approval. It also means that remedies that have FDA approval may not be safe and effective, since drug companies have been known to skew their research results and withhold information about side effects.[9] Even when no one is at fault, serious side effects are often revealed only after years of widespread use.[10]

Natural remedies for women's complaints that we'll be looking at in this book include herbal remedies and natural hormones. These remedies are safe and effective; but because they are not FDA-approved, manufacturers must be cautious in their claims. Natural hormone products must keep such a low profile that even if you see them on store shelves, you may not know what they are. The labels on the available natural progesterone creams, for example, nowhere say "progesterone." Instead, they use terms like "moisturizing cream" and "wild yam extract." Why? Because if they were labeled "progesterone," they would run the risk of being classified as drugs by the FDA. The Food, Drug, and Cosmetic Act allows the FDA broad powers to regulate "articles intended for use in the diagnosis, cure, mitigation, treatment, or prevention of disease in man or other animals;" and "articles (other than food) intended to affect the structure or any function of the body of man or other animals." To fall outside this definition, a product must either have no health-promoting benefits or be a food. (There is an interesting anomaly here. Cigarettes and alcohol are not subject to FDA regulation because they don't pretend to be good for your health. Only healthful products that will or might prevent or cure disease must undergo extensive and expensive testing before sale.)

The only "progesterones" that are clearly labeled or well known are the patentable synthetics. Unfortunately, these are also the varieties that can have serious side effects. Hormones work like keys in a lock. The slightest variation in the key can prevent it from performing its intended functions. Since patented drugs *cannot* be exact replicas of the body's own hormones, they cannot be exact copies of the "key." That makes them both less safe and less effective than their cheaper natural counterparts, which can be exact replicas of human hormones. Plants make molecules that are the precursors of human progesterone and that can easily be converted to it.[12]

Due to FDA strictures, however, natural plant hormones are a well-kept secret, promoted only by that handful of practitioners who have used them and seen how well they work on their patients. One of these practitioners is Lynne Walker, a doctor of pharmacy, licensed acupuncturist, doctor of homeopathy, and consulting co-author of this book.

Dr. Walker broadened her interests from pharmacy to holistic medicine when, at the age of thirty-three, she was told that she needed a hysterectomy due to a large fibroid tumor in her uterus. Before she agreed to surgery, she went to Linda Forbes, an acupuncturist and chiropractor practicing in Santa Monica, California, who gave her Chinese herbs and homeopathic remedies. When these resolved Dr. Walker's problem without surgery, she was so impressed that she went on to study Chinese medicine at Emperor's College and homeopathy at the British Institute of Homeopathy in Santa Monica, from which she obtained a Doctor of Homeopathy degree. Since then she has helped women with a wide range of hormone-related symptoms, both in her private practice as an acupuncturist and as a pharmacist at a holistic drugstore.

I met Dr. Walker in the office of Dr. Forbes. I was then a full-time attorney and mother of two young children, seeking to revive my flagging energy. Dr. Forbes' remedies helped me deal with the stresses I was under. I now live abroad with my family, where I have time to research and write in the health field; and since I am in it, the subject of menopause particularly interests me at the moment. Before I got "hooked" on estrogen, I decided to delve into the studies. This book looks at those studies, which were not reassuring, and at research on the less well known natural remedies that Dr. Walker has found in her practice to be safer and more effective for menopausal and premenstrual complaints.

—Ellen Hodgson Brown
Tegucigalpa, Honduras
October 1993

I.

Hormone Replacement: Another Look

Chapter One

Was It Really Supposed to Be This Way?

What is the prime of life? May it not be defined as a period of about twenty years in a woman's life, and thirty in a man's?

—Plato, *The Republic*

At forty-three, Joan left a responsible position with the IRS to take on the challenge of computerizing Kenya's tax system. She had a new husband and was enthusiastic about her new career in an exotic country.

Joan had always tried to take care of herself, eating right and getting regular exercise. But lately her health routine hadn't been working for her. She was tired, nervous, anxious, even distraught. Foods that never used to bother her upset her stomach. When other people were cold, she was dripping in sweat. Her husband was supportive, but she was losing her interest in sex; and she wondered how he could be interested, since she felt she looked old and drawn.

On top of that, she could no longer cope with her work. Aggravations that never used to bother her now drove her over the edge. When things finally got so bad that she consulted a doctor, she half-expected him to say he was going to have to send her to the United States and institutionalize her for a little rest. "That's fine, I understand," she would reply. Instead, he told her about the Change of Life and the problems caused by erratic hormones. His solution was to put her on estrogen.

The drug marvelously transformed her outlook on life. Unfortunately, it also aggravated her uterine fibroid tumors. In the end, she submitted to surgery and had her uterus removed.

Joan's roller coaster ride with menopause is not an unusual case. Symptoms common to modern menopausal women include not only hot flashes and loss of interest in sex but depression, moodiness, crying, anger, irritability, shortness of breath or difficult breathing, dizziness, fatigue, indigestion, constipation, diarrhea, gas, headaches, heart palpitations, night sweats, insomnia, muscle and bone aches and tingling, shoulder and hip pain, cramps in the legs and feet, numbness in the arms, painfully sensitive skin, urinary problems, memory loss and mental sluggishness, dryness of the skin and vaginal tissues, breast tenderness and weight gain.

Hot flashes are not usually the first symptoms of menopause, but they are its hallmark. When you've had one, you know you're in menopause. Hot flashes are suffered by more than two-thirds of women and are the most common reason they seek medical attention for menopausal complaints. Eighty percent of these women endure hot flashes for more than a year, and twenty-five to fifty percent suffer them for more than five years. For a few they can drag on for ten years or more.

"It's not easy looking cool and confident," complained Liz, a Los Angeles attorney, "when my face is red as a beet and covered in sweat. And it generally happens when I need to look authoritative, like when I'm arguing in court. But the nights are the worst. Ten minutes after I fall asleep, I wake up in a cold sweat. It may take a whole hour to get back to sleep, and ten minutes later I'm awake again in a sweat. I'm up half the night. Needless to say, it's hard to be at my best the next day."

Hot flashes were once thought to be psychosomatic, an emotional reaction to that time of life when a woman's children had left home and she wasn't sure what to do with herself. But recent studies have shown (as women themselves knew all along) that hot flashes are very real physiological events. Sweating and a rise in skin temperature have been directly tied to a pulsating surge in the production of luteinizing hormone (LH), the hormone responsible for stimulating

the egg follicles to secrete estrogen. Apparently, as hormone production drops off at menopause, LH secretion increases in an attempt
to squeeze the last drops from a dry well. The result can be a radical
fluctuation in body temperature.[1]

Was it really supposed to be this way? Not according to African
researcher Llaila Afrika, who pointed out in *African Holistic Health*
that the menopausal symptoms of Western women aren't common
among women in other cultures eating natural diets and following
holistic lifestyles. Studies show that Japanese women rarely experience hot flushes and other menopausal symptoms.[2] Mayan women
have virtually no menopausal complaints.[3] Women in certain non-
Western countries also manage to escape the degenerative diseases
that plague American senior citizens: heart disease, cancer, and osteoporosis.[4] How do they do it, and why can't we?

Nature seems to have intended menopause to be a gradual process
of reduced hormone output by the ovaries. The ovaries belong to a
complex of glands known as the steroid glands that includes the testes
and adrenal cortex. All of them are under the control of the pituitary. As ovarian function falls off and hormone levels drop, the pituitary sends signals to the adrenals to increase their hormone output.
What was lost from the ovaries is then partly replaced by these glands.
The adrenal glands increase their estrogen output naturally with age
in both sexes. They can secrete substantial amounts of it not only
after menopause but after hysterectomy, even with the ovaries
removed.

When this backup hormone system is working properly, the
Change should come with few or no side effects. Chinese doctors say
that your flow should stop without symptoms at around the age of
fifty-six—the later the better, since menstruation is considered an
internal cleansing process. Why doesn't this backup system work for
us? The blame has been put on adrenal exhaustion, caused by stress,
low blood sugar, and poor diet.

Recent research suggests that a natural plant-based diet can compensate to some extent for hormone deficiencies. Plants, like animals, contain hormones that regulate cell metabolism and growth.
Some plant foods contain substantial amounts of the sterols that are

the precursors of human estrogen and progesterone. Soy products such as tofu, miso, soybeans, and boiled beans have particularly high amounts of these sterols. Their abundance in the Oriental diet helps explain the notable lack of menopausal complaints among Japanese women.[5] The Oriental diet also differs from ours in being low in animal fat, which suppresses progesterone production. We'll explore these dietary mechanisms later.

Hormone levels are also depressed by stress. To understand the reason requires an understanding of the interrelationships of the steroid hormones. The steroid glands produce about thirty known hormones from the cholesterol distributed throughout the body. These hormones are of five types:

1. *Estrogens* (estrone, estradiol, estriol) are primarily produced by the ovarian follicles. They maintain female secondary characteristics.

2. *Androgens* (testosterone, androsterone) are typical products of the testes. They maintain male secondary characteristics.

3. *Gestagens* (i.e. progesterone) are released by the ovary's corpus luteum, the "yellow body" that remains after an egg is released. They maintain pregnancy.

4. *Glucocorticoids* (e.g. cortisol and its precursor cortisone) are products of the adrenal cortex. They transform proteins into glucose, causing blood sugar to rise. Cortisol is the adrenal hormone responsible for "fight or flight."

5. *Mineralocorticoids* (e.g. aldosterone) maintain mineral and water balance.

The two major hormones produced by the ovaries are estrogen and progesterone. Estrogen builds up the endometrium (the lining of the uterus) in preparation for supporting a developing fetus. It does this by proliferating endometrial cells into a thickened tissue. Progesterone is released after the ovary drops an egg into the fallopian tube, about two weeks into the monthly cycle. It prepares the lining of the uterus to nurture a fertilized egg. If the egg isn't fertilized, progesterone breaks down the thickened endometrial lining into layers ready to be shed.

Progesterone, however, has other important functions. It's the precursor to all the other steroid hormones, including not only estrogen

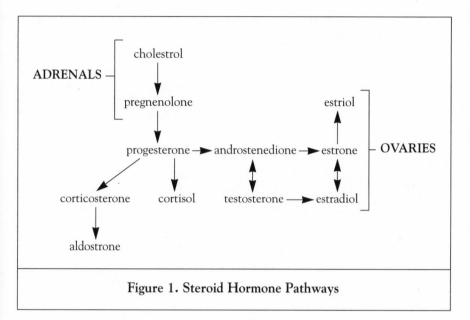

Figure 1. Steroid Hormone Pathways

but cortisol, the "fight or flight" hormone. These interrelated hormone pathways are shown in Figure 1. When you're under stress, your progesterone is converted to cortisol at the expense of the progesterone and estrogen necessary for specifically female functions. The result is hormone deficiency. This deficiency is particularly troublesome at menopause, when hormone production is already rapidly declining. Stress has been shown in laboratory studies to increase the frequency of hot flashes.[6]

Chapter Two

A Question of Balance

The superior doctor prevents illness; the mediocre doctor cures imminent illness; the inferior doctor treats illness.

—Chinese proverb

The same stress syndrome that explains the more severe menopausal symptoms of Western women can explain the greater prevalence of premenstrual syndrome today than when our mothers were young. More women are trying to juggle a job and a family. Our stress levels are up and our female hormone levels are down. Our progesterone is being converted to cortisol at the expense of the hormones required for specifically female functions.

PMS: When hormones start to fail

Premenstrual syndrome (PMS) is a symptom complex that can include headaches, abdominal bloating, breast swelling, fluid retention, increased thirst, increased appetite, cravings for sweet or salty foods, and emotional symptoms including anxiety, irritability, mood swings, depression, hostility, crying, and loss of self-confidence. PMS sets in seven to ten days before a woman starts her period. The condition normally begins sometime in the thirties, when hormone production is slowing down.

Connie's was the extreme case. "I was too irritable to speak or be spoken to in the morning," she recalls, "and it did not get better as the day went on. I was in an almost constant state of teeth-clench-

9

ing aggravation. I kept it hidden, but not very well. I had difficulty speaking in a civil tone to my teenage children. In fact, when I was at home, I rarely had a good word about anything. Normal occurrences or minor annoyances often sent me into such a rage, I had to hide by myself for fear someone would witness these ugly emotions going on inside me. I thought of myself as a person with super-human self-control because I did not give in to the extremely violent images and urges raging inside me. The week or so before my period, self-control went out the window. I honestly believed at times that I was crazy. My normal state of agitation gave way to mood swings ranging from deep depression to episodes of screaming, ranting, and fits of violence. Self-loathing intensified these feelings. At times, I would cry for hours on end for no apparent reason."

Like hot flashes, premenstrual symptoms like these were once thought to be psychosomatic. Then in the fifties, British gynecologist Katharina Dalton found that nearly half the women admitted to a hospital for accidents or psychological illnesses were in their premenstrual week. Other studies showed that about half the crimes for which women were responsible were committed during this period.[1] (These studies looked good for PMS but bad for equal employment, since employers began to question whether women were stable hires; but other investigations showed that women performed as well intellectually in the throes of PMS as otherwise.) PMS is now thought to plague from 25 to 90 percent of all women, depending on how it is defined.

Dr. Dalton was personally interested because she, too, was a victim. She was a chronic sufferer of premenstrual migraine headaches. Then she noticed that her symptoms went away during the last six months of her pregnancy. Progesterone levels are twenty to thirty times higher then than at other times. Surmising a link, she proceeded to treat herself with daily progesterone injections after her baby was born. Her migraines did not come back. She published her first reports in 1953. Thousands of women with PMS have been successfully treated with natural progesterone since.[2]

One of these treatment successes was Connie, the woman who cried for no apparent reason. The first time she used natural progesterone, she cried again; but this time she knew why she was crying.

"I cried for all those lost years since adolescence. Because within ten minutes of applying the [natural progesterone] cream, I experienced a calm I never thought possible for me. I cried because I realized for the first time that I was not an evil person." Four months after starting on this natural hormone, she reported that her relationship with her husband and children had become "a joy instead of a burden." A number of other physical problems unexpectedly cleared up, including migraine headaches, frequent nosebleeds, tooth-grinding, leg aches and cramps, poor circulation, dark spots on her face, insomnia, poor complexion, and menstrual cramps.

We'll look at this and other hormone-restoring remedies in detail later. What we want to consider here is what these cases tell us about PMS. Why would natural progesterone relieve the condition?

Researchers say that during the normal menstrual cycle, immediately after ovulation, levels of both estrogen and progesterone rise, and they continue to rise until menstruation. The progesterone acts as an estrogen antagonist. It keeps estrogen levels from going too high. But progesterone stores can be depleted by stress—emotional, dietary, or environmental. Stress, as we've seen, causes progesterone to be converted to cortisol. Without enough progesterone, estrogen levels get too high.

Excess estrogen can then produce symptoms associated with PMS, including salt and fluid retention, low blood sugar, blood clotting, breast tenderness, thyroid problems, and weight gain.[3] All of these symptoms are listed as side effects in the package inserts for prescription estrogen. These physical imbalances produce the mood swings and other psychological effects that women associate with PMS. Progesterone can correct them by normalizing estrogen levels.

Oddly, these symptoms of excess estrogen sound very much like those attributed to *insufficient* estrogen at menopause. Hormone researcher Raymond F. Peat, professor of biochemistry at Blake College in Oregon, explains both syndromes as due to a progesterone deficiency.[4] While estrogen levels do drop at menopause, progesterone levels can drop even more. For estrogen to be dominant, huge amounts aren't necessary if progesterone isn't being produced to oppose it; and that is the case at perimenopause.

Progesterone is dependent on ovulation. It comes from the corpus luteum, the piece of egg follicle that is left behind after an egg is released. During perimenopause, though you are still having monthly periods, you are often not dropping eggs. That means progesterone is not being produced, leaving estrogen dominant. The result can be the symptoms of estrogen excess that typically afflict women around the Change.

Hormones and cancer

Depressed progesterone levels can also be responsible for the endometrial cancers and possibly the breast cancers prevalent at menopause. Estrogen is known to stimulate the growth of tumors, and progesterone checks this growth.[5]

Estrogen's principal function is cellular proliferation and growth. "Estrogen is the hormone for beginnings," says Dr. Peat, "a sort of biochemical eraser which can eliminate recently recorded information, restoring the underlying primitive capacity for growth."[6]

Primitive growth characterizes not only the fetus but the proliferation of cells known as cancer. In 1902, John Beard, a professor of embryology at the University of Edinburgh in Scotland, published a paper in the British medical journal *The Lancet* showing that there was no detectable difference between highly malignant cancer cells and certain pre-embryonic cells that are normal to the early stages of pregnancy. Most of these normal pre-embryonic cells are found in the ovaries or testes, but some are distributed elsewhere in the body, where they are thought to be involved in regenerating damaged or aging tissue. Wherever the body is damaged, estrogen is also found in great concentrations in both men and women. It seems to serve as a stimulus to cellular growth and repair.[7]

"When we are threatened, by injury or aging," states Dr. Peat, "we need the capacity for renewal of cells."[8] Most primary tumors occur where there is cell renewal due to irritation or trauma. Cancer results when the normal regenerative growth gets out of control; and progesterone helps keep it under control. Progesterone has been shown to cause the regression of tumors induced by estrogen.[9]

In his book *Nutrition for Women*, Dr. Peat explains that estrogen

12

and progesterone are antagonists in many ways. They have opposite metabolic effects and act to balance each other in the body. Estrogen causes salt and fluid retention, lowers blood sugar, opposes thyroxin (the principal thyroid hormone), and promotes blood clotting. Progesterone has the reverse effect in each case. Estrogen increases the risk of embolisms, uterine fibroids, high blood pressure, fibrocystic breasts, and cancer of the breast and endometrium. Again, progesterone has the reverse effect in each case.[10] In the bones, estrogen inhibits the osteoclasts, the cells that tear down old bone. Progesterone stimulates the osteoblasts, the cells that make new bone.[11]

Another hormone involved in this system of checks and balances is thyroid hormone. The thyroid gland, located at the base of the neck in front, furnishes energy to every cell in the body, and its functions are linked to progesterone. Both thyroid and progesterone regulate metabolism, normalize and de-stress the pituitary, oppose the effects of stress, aid nutrition, and are blocked by stress and promoted by good nutrition. Stress releases cortisone, which inhibits the thyroid and causes a rise in estrogen levels and a drop in thyroid and progesterone levels. Estrogen impairs the action of thyroid, while progesterone enhances it.[12] Women taking estrogen supplements often complain of chronic fatigue or lack of energy, symptoms of hypothyroidism. When thyroid tests are found to be normal, the symptoms are ascribed to old age. But if natural progesterone is given to these women, their symptoms disappear.[13]

Excess estrogen impedes cellular respiration, while progesterone and thyroid hormone both have the opposite effect. In research which won the Nobel Prize in the thirties, Otto Warburg demonstrated that all cancer involves defective cellular respiration. The theory helps explain why estrogen is linked to cancer. It also suggests that natural progesterone and thyroid hormone, which improve cellular respiration, could be useful in the treatment of cancer. Clinical experience has shown this to be true.[14]

Balancing hormones

Debate continues over whether a shortage of estrogen or of progesterone causes menopausal symptoms. The answer may be different for different women. A similar uncertainty revolves around the symptoms of PMS, since estrogen levels in PMS sufferers have been found to be either higher, lower, or substantially the same as in women without symptoms.[15] Fortunately, to use the natural remedies we'll be looking at in this book, one does not need to know the answers to these questions. The remedies work, not by replacing lost hormones with synthetics, but by stimulating the body to correct its own hormone imbalances.

In the case of hot flashes, imbalance, not hormone shortage, actually produces symptoms. If hot flashes were due to a shortage of estrogen, women should have worse hot flashes in their seventies (when estrogen levels are lower) than in their fifties. Why isn't this the case? Symptoms result, apparently, not from a shortage, but when the pituitary is adjusting the thermostat in an effort to get hormone levels back on an even keel.

Chinese and Western herbal, homeopathic, and natural hormonal remedies help the body correct imbalances without distressing symptoms. Each of these natural therapeutic approaches has its own diagnostic system for determining the appropriate remedy to nudge the body back into balance. The advantage of this approach is that you avoid overdosing on a hormone you may not need, exposing yourself to side effects and long-term risks. If the body is given the right raw materials—proper food, vitamins, and minerals—it can make what it needs.

The Western approach to alleviating menopausal symptoms is to replace our missing hormones with synthetic or semi-synthetic pharmaceutical substitutes; but this approach has serious drawbacks. Before we get to the alternatives, let's take a closer look at the trials of modern Western women around the Change and at the problems with the conventional approaches to solving them.

Chapter Three

Menopause and the Drug Revolution

For fifty years the ritual has been the same. Every winter, they strap a diaper-like apparatus on their pregnant mares and collect the horses' urine. Periodically, a truck from Wyeth-Ayerst Laboratories picks up the urine. The company extracts and refines a hormone from it used to produce Premarin, a popular drug that treats such postmenopausal symptoms as hot flashes.

—*The Philadelphia Inquirer* (March 1993)[1]

The pharmaceutical industry's response to the loss of hormones at menopause was supplemental hormones either extracted from animals or made in the laboratory.

In the United States, the most popular oral estrogen is Ayerst's Premarin. Ayerst advertises that it has dispensed 25 billion tablets of the drug, currently priced at 36 cents a tablet. Premarin is derived from pregnant mare's urine, as is its name. That makes it a "natural" product; but it's really *natural* only to horses. The urine of horses contains equilin and other estrogens not normally found in humans. Because they don't have the same molecular structure as human estrogens (estrone, estradiol, and estriol), they can't be used by human estrogen receptors. Oral Premarin produces blood levels of equilin that are many times higher than those of estradiol or estrone.[2]

Further, because Premarin is an oral pill, it must first pass through the stomach and liver, where much of the dose is lost to digestion.

Larger doses than those found naturally in the bloodstream are therefore required, potentially increasing side effects and risks. Adverse
reactions to Premarin listed in the *Physician's Desk Reference* (*PDR*),
the standard medical reference on drugs, include PMS-like symptoms; breast tenderness, enlargement and secretion; nausea, vomit-
ing, abdominal cramps and bloating; skin and eye sensitivities;
headaches, dizziness and depression; weight gain and water retention; bleeding between periods or missed periods; changes in libido
(sex drive); and enlargement of uterine fibroid tumors.

Like estrogen, progesterone was originally obtained from animals.
At the turn of the century, menopause was treated with corpus luteum
(the part of the ovary that produces progesterone) extracted from
sows. Then in 1934, pure progesterone was isolated from the sow's
corpus luteum and its chemical structure was determined. Reports
were soon published of its beneficial effects in cases of miscarriage,
arthritis, infertility, cancer, and diseases of the nervous system. However, this crystalline progesterone could not be taken in pill form
because it was converted by the liver and excreted too rapidly to be
absorbed into the bloodstream. It had to be injected, a process that
was cumbersome, expensive, and ran the risk of toxic debris left at
the injection site. Another problem with this pure progesterone was
that it was generic material in the public domain that could not be
patented. Interest in it therefore waned, as the drug industry found
ways to convert it into patentable synthetic forms of steroid hormones—progestins, estrogens, and glucocorticoids.[3]

The estrogens that continued to be most popular for menopausal
complaints were those derived from horses. Side effects notwith-
standing, Premarin seemed for many women to be a wonder drug. It
eliminated their hot flashes, and it revived their lost interest in sex.
Estrogen replacement therapy (ERT) was also linked to a reduction
in the risk of heart disease and osteoporosis. In many ways, it looked
like the fountain of youth prophesied by Dr. Wilson.

There were, however, grounds for pause. By 1947, when DES, a
synthetic estrogen, became popular to prevent miscarriage, over three
hundred papers had been written indicating that estrogen causes cancer in animals. These warnings went unheeded, as DES continued

Menopause and the Drug Revolution

ers have estrogenic effects. They can bring on fluid retention and edema (swelling), symptoms related to an excess of estrogen.

There is also the inconvenience that 85 percent of women taking progestins continue to have monthly bleeding (along with 25 percent of women on estrogen alone). The other negative side effects come just before this bleeding, or in the "premenstrual" phase. They're similar to the symptoms of PMS except they're drug-induced. (They're called "iatrogenic" PMS.) Some of these side effects can be avoided by switching progestins, since different brands are more or less androgenic. But all of them have side effects. With the androgenic types (Norlutin, Norlutate), you get acne and greasy skin and hair. With the estrogenic types (Provera, Amen), you get depression and anxiety.[10]

These drawbacks have resulted in a compliance problem for doctors: many women either can't or won't take prescription hormones. Robert Rebar, M.D., at the University of Cincinnati (Ohio) College of Medicine, reports that two-thirds of the women who start on estrogen replacement therapy at his university's clinic wind up abandoning the pursuit.[11]

Women who can tolerate estrogen are liable to give up HRT because of the progestin they have to take with it for half the month. Other women would like to take hormones but have been told by their doctors that they can't.

Women who can't take estrogen

ERT is contraindicated for women with a family history or prior diagnosis of breast cancer, fibroids (benign tumors on the wall of the uterus), asthma, migraine headaches, epilepsy, heart or kidney disease, gallstones, stroke, high blood pressure, thrombosis, pulmonary blockage, and undiagnosed abnormal genital bleeding.

Noreen is one of these women. The wife of an ambassador, her major official function is entertaining. Often it's the stress of coordinating huge official functions that brings on her hot flashes. She finds herself greeting her guests bathed in sweat. She took estrogen for awhile, but it made her breasts so sensitive that she couldn't stand even her clothing brushing against them; and then she had a Pap smear suggesting cervical cancer. Her doctors treated her with drugs (causing her to lose most of her lush auburn hair), then said she should studiously avoid ERT. That means she is denied even this Hobson's choice.

Normal women without contraindications may also have to suffer for long periods without the benefit of hormones, since most doctors no longer consider estrogen to be safe until after a woman has quit having periods of any sort.[12]

Virginia is a 52-year-old British expatriate who started having hot flashes long before her doctor would give her estrogen. Normally prim and proper, she recalls the day her husband came home to find her lying naked on the bed, frantically waving her legs at the ceiling fan. "What the hell are you doing?" he asked. "I'm so-o-o hot!" was all she could reply.

Virginia would have welcomed medical relief; but her doctor said that taking hormones while she was still having monthly periods was not safe, since her body might already be producing huge amounts of estrogen in an effort to get her ovaries working again.

Even when your doctor says it's safe to take estrogen, you may have trouble finding a comfortable dose. The appropriate amount of estrogen for your body can change from day to day as hormone production changes. A worse problem is that increasing your estrogen intake raises the "set-point" below which your pituitary reacts with hot flashes. When you try to stop taking the hormone, you can wind up with more devastating hot flashes than the ones you started out with.

Heather wasn't suffering serious menopausal symptoms when her doctor put her on estrogen, so she wasn't prepared for the crippling hot flashes and anxiety attacks that hit her when she tried to quit taking it. Now she's back on the drug. In effect, she has developed a dependence on estrogen.

Many women, knowing their discomfort will only be temporary, would be persuaded by these drawbacks to endure their hot flashes like their grandmothers did, without help. But these same women are likely to be launched down the hormone path by the fear of consequences that are more serious and irreversible—heart disease and osteoporosis.

Chapter Four

Cancer, Heart Disease, and Osteoporosis: Are We Trading One Disease for Another?

How do we know that estrogen prevents heart disease? We don't have a single prospective study.

—Wulf H. Utian, president of the
North American Menopause Society (1992)[1]

Probably the last, strongest argument for the widespread use of estrogen is that it supposedly delays the development of osteoporosis. The absence of osteoporosis in old women in many other countries is never discussed in the professional meetings on osteoporosis subsidized by the drug companies.

—Hormone researcher Ray Peat[2]

Today, women who aren't afraid of hot flashes may be propelled into hormone replacement by a more frightening prospect: the irreversible bone loss and cardiovascular disease that experts say are the long-term consequences of estrogen deprivation. That's what some experts say, but others worry that the benefits are uncertain and that the trade-off is an increased risk of cancer.

Although cardiovascular disease is the number one cause of death in the United States,[3] breast cancer now takes the lives of more women in the menopausal years between thirty-seven and fifty-five than any other disease; and according to the Centers for Disease Control and Prevention, the United States is on the verge of a marked increase as the Baby Boomers enter this age group.[4]

The Nurses' Health Study was a massive long-term study involving 121,700 female registered nurses. It looked at both breast cancer and heart disease risk, providing a rare opportunity to compare risks and benefits in the same group of women. A review of the two reports, published in the medical journal *Family Practice* in 1991, concluded:

> From these two studies one can estimate that as compared to never-users, the risk of a coronary event in current hormone users was reduced from 1.12 to 0.36 per 10,000 person years. In contrast the risk of breast cancer increased from 18.99 to 23.79 per 10,000 person years.[5]

Even if the trade were an even one, some women might prefer a quick heart attack in their beds to a lengthy and excruciating cancer; but the odds weren't that good. The risk of breast cancer even for never-users was seventeen times as great as the risk of a coronary event (non-fatal myocardial infarction or fatal coronary heart disease), and approximately five new breast cancer cases resulted for every one coronary event that was prevented on hormone therapy.

The FDA has never approved HRT for use as hormone replacement therapy in menopausal women.[6] While this sounds shocking, it is actually normal in the trade. "Crude estimates are that unapproved uses account for at least one-fourth of all prescriptions," explains former Federal Trade Commission agent John Calfee. "The FDA approves new drugs only for specified applications ... but physicians are free to prescribe approved drugs for any use ... These new uses are almost never submitted for FDA approval, because the millions of dollars and years of effort needed for a second approval cannot be justified for a drug whose patent life has already been abbreviated by the original lengthy approval process."[7]

The *Family Practice* reviewers concluded of HRT, "The effect of combined estrogen and progesterone therapy on the risk of breast cancer is unknown."[8] What is known is that the incidence of the disease has gone up by more than thirty percent since the seventies, when this hormone combination became popular.

"Millions of postmenopausal women are currently being treated with drug therapies whose long-term effects are not adequately known," says Wulf H. Utian, Director of the Department of Obstetrics and Gynecology at the University Hospitals of Cleveland and president of the North American Menopause Society. "It's scandalous that we don't yet have the answers we need."[9]

The studies on this point are technical, but we want to go into them in detail because the issue is important and highly controversial.

The heart disease controversy

Doctors recommending estrogen for heart disease rely on studies showing that women taking estrogen have a lower rate of the disease than women not taking it, and that estrogen lowers low-density lipoprotein (LDL or "bad") cholesterol and raises high-density lipoprotein (HDL or "good") cholesterol.[10]

But other experts observe that the reduction in heart disease deaths proposed for estrogen still hasn't been proven in a randomized trial.[11] A randomized trial is one in which women are selected at random to be in either the drug group or the non-drug group, then watched for developments. This protocol avoids biases of self-selection, in which women who are already less healthy and more likely to die early tend to avoid hormone replacement (since they have a higher risk of cancer and other unwanted side effects), while women who are more healthy and likely to live longer tend to opt for the hormones. Studies cited as proving that estrogen prevents heart disease may prove only that women who are less likely to get heart disease tend to take estrogen.

This bias could explain the results of one of the most encouraging studies for HRT to date. In a British study reported in 1990, deaths among 4,544 longterm HRT users were less than half those expected in the general population, not only from heart disease but from all causes. However, this wasn't the result you would expect if the low death rate were due to the known biological effects of the drugs on serum cholesterol. The observed effect should have been mainly on heart disease deaths; but low mortality was seen in nearly all causes of death. Disturbingly, in a followup study, one of the few risks to increase for the women on HRT was for breast cancer. The finding suggested an adverse effect which took time to show up in a basically healthy, low-risk population.[12]

Even in estrogen trials that haven't been randomized, findings have been inconsistent. Consider two studies reported in the same issue of the *New England Journal of Medicine* in 1985. One was an early report of the Nurses' Health Study. It found that women who had used estrogen had only about half the risk of contracting coronary disease as other women, while those who were currently using it had only about a third the risk.[13] In the Framingham Study reported in the same issue, however, estrogen users had a more than fifty percent *greater* risk of contracting coronary disease than non-users.[14] The Framingham Study researchers explained the discrepancies by suggesting that their assessment was more complete than in other studies and that women who use postmenopausal therapy tend to have fewer risk factors for heart disease than non-users.[15]

Women with high blood pressure are sometimes put on estrogen to *protect* their hearts, but in the Framingham Study, estrogen users were found to have significantly higher blood pressure than non-users. They also had twice the risk of cerebrovascular disease (stroke). The fear of stroke is a major reason women worry about their blood pressures.

Some other studies have also found higher blood pressures in women using estrogen.[16] The package insert for prescription estrogen warns, "Taking estrogens may cause ... the blood to clot more easily, possibly allowing clots to form in your bloodstream. If blood clots do form in your bloodstream, they can cut off the blood supply to vital organs, causing serious problems. These problems may include a stroke (by cutting off blood to the brain) [or] a heart attack (by cutting off blood to the heart). ... "

"The billion-dollar estrogen industry has learned the trick of directing the public's attention to where some plausible benefit might be expected," observes Dr. Peat, "and of politely ignoring the areas where death and destruction are in fact being produced."[17] He points out that the greatest *downside* of oral contraceptives—which also contain estrogens—is generally considered to be their *increased* risk of heart disease; and that when estrogen has been used experimentally to prevent heart attacks in men, it actually induced them. Estrogen causes a magnesium deficiency, which promotes clotting and abnormal fat metabolism. Numerous studies link a magnesium deficiency to heart disease.[18]

Even if the cardiovascular benefits of estrogen were firmly established, there would be the problem that its favorable effects on HDL (good) cholesterol seem to be reversed when progestins accompany it. Harmful lipoprotein changes resulting from progestins have been enough in some studies to actually increase heart disease risk.[19] (That's not true, however, for *natural* progesterone, as we'll see later.)

Besides cancer and blood clots, risks accompanying ERT include damage to the liver and gallbladder. To get enough estrogen into the bloodstream to lower cholesterol, it needs to be taken orally. That means it passes through the digestive system and the liver, where it can create benign tumors and can overstimulate the gallbladder, increasing your risk of gallstones by a factor of two or three.[20]

These problems are eliminated with the transdermal estrogen patch (Estraderm), which avoids digestion by delivering estrogen through the skin. However, absorption from the patch is variable, being most rapid when first applied. Some doctors feel it offers inconsistent amounts of the hormone, making its effects on cholesterol levels and bone preservation unreliable. The patch is less likely than oral estrogen to increase your level of HDL (good) cholesterol. Oral HRT is the only therapy recommended by most doctors if your main goal is prevention of heart disease. Both oral preparations and the patch may cause breast tenderness and changes in the cells lining the uterus, so both may increase cancer risk.[21]

Even if estrogen lowers heart disease risk, there may be ways of getting the same result without exposing yourself to cancer and other side effects. A 1990 University of Tennessee study found there was indeed a link between estrogen and lowered coronary artery disease deaths—but *only in women who already had the disease*. In women with normal coronary vessels, estrogen benefits were insignificant.[22] That means if you have normal, healthy arteries, you're incurring risks without benefits by taking estrogen. Your arteries can be safely kept normal and healthy through proper diet and exercise. (See Chapter Fourteen.)

The osteoporosis epidemic

The other postmenopausal threat underlying the estrogen craze is osteoporosis, or age-related bone loss. The problem is a serious one, but some researchers question whether estrogen is the solution.

Osteoporosis causes an estimated 1.3 million fractures annually in the United States, at a national cost approaching $10 billion. The most damaging consequences are hip fractures. They occur nearly seven times as frequently in elderly women as in elderly men. Each year, 60,000 women die within six months of their fractures, and the numbers are going up. For the survivors, hip fractures can mean living out life at a nursing home, where they are the second most common cause of admission.[23] Many women are at risk: those who have a low vitamin D and calcium intake, a family history of osteoporosis (fractures or rounding of the upper back), an early menopause or hysterectomy/oophorectomy, lower than average levels of male hormones; those who have never been pregnant, are small and thin (since fat-soluble hormones are stored in body fat), inactive, northern European, light-skinned and light-haired, coffee or alcohol drinkers, or on cortisone therapy.

Bone loss takes a dramatic jump when hormone secretion falls off at menopause, up to 1.5 percent or more per year. Adding estrogen seems to slow it down. "There is evidence that bone loss is increased in many women following the menopause," says the *PDR*, "but there is no clear way to identify those women who will develop osteoporotic fractures. There is also evidence that the rate of bone loss can be reduced in postmenopausal women by taking estrogens. . . . " The wholesale prescription of estrogen has resulted from this uncertainty concerning who will be victims.

But estrogen is an imperfect solution. The prescription package insert concedes, "There is no evidence that estrogen replacement therapy restores bone mass to premenopausal levels." It merely slows down bone loss; and the dose necessary to do this is higher than you need to control other postmenopausal symptoms, further increasing cancer risk.[24] Moreover, to keep receiving estrogen's benefits, you have to keep taking it for life. Researchers have found that within four years of discontinuing ERT, there was no detectable difference in bone mineral content between women who had never taken the drug and those who began treatment but gave it up.[25]

On the other hand, even if you keep taking estrogen, it may not keep preventing bone loss. A 1988 review in the *American Journal of Medicine* concluded that "in postmenopausal women with established osteoporosis, hormonal therapy, alone or with vitamin D metabolites and calcium supplements, may not be of significant benefit, and may be associated with a high rate of unacceptable side effects and complications." It concluded that "administration of this hormone six years or more after menopause may no longer be effective."[26]

There are better, more natural alternatives, as we'll see in Section II.

The cancer threat

For its uncertain benefits to the heart and the bones, women who take estrogen trade an increased risk of a disease whose magnitude is already ominous. Each year in the United States, there are 180,000 new breast cancer cases and 46,000 deaths. Another 150,000 women undergo mutilating mastectomies. Breast cancer incidence has gone up more than three percent a year every year since 1980. It now strikes one in nine women sometime in their lives. In 1992, breast cancer claimed 327,000 years of potential life, assuming an average life expectancy of sixty-five.[27]

Estrogen is well known to stimulate breast tumors in animals, and the same effect is strongly suggested by human studies.[28] But researchers had hoped that adding synthetic progestins would counter the risk of breast cancer as it does for endometrial cancer. Unfortunately, most studies haven't borne this out. In fact the *PDR* says Provera *causes* breast malignancies in beagle dogs.[29]

A Swedish study reported in 1989 found that in women taking the estrogen/progestin combination, breast cancer risk actually quadrupled. By contrast, women taking estrogen alone had only a modestly increased risk.[30] This finding "hits at the heart of our philosophy that patients should be on estrogen and progestin," said Dr. Jonathan S. Berek, Director of Gynecologic Oncology at the UCLA School of Medicine. "This questions the assumption that it is entirely safe, at

27

least from the standpoint of the breast."[31]

The Swedish study has been criticized because the number of patients actually completing it was small (196 out of 23,000 women receiving questionnaires). However, in September of 1992, the same trend was confirmed in a twelve-year followup of the massive Nurses' Health Study, involving 121,700 women. Women currently using estrogen and progestins together were found to be one and a half times as likely to contract breast cancer as women never using hormones, while women currently using progestins alone were found to be two and a half times as likely to contract the disease.[32] Like the Swedish study, the Nurses' Study proved the reverse of what had been hoped—that progestins would counter estrogen's increased risk of breast cancer, as they do for endometrial cancer. The researchers distinguished the contrary findings of an often-cited earlier study by Gambrell and associates on grounds that it involved a smaller number of cases and was not adjusted for age.[33]

Even for estrogen alone, the breast cancer risk for nurses who were current estrogen users was found to be 42 percent greater than for never-users. This finding was also contrary to some earlier studies. A 1991 review of earlier studies concluded that menopausal therapy consisting of 0.625 mg/dl or less of conjugated estrogens does not increase breast cancer risk.[34]

Why the difference? The researchers studying the nurses pointed out that most previous studies did not distinguish current from past estrogen use, and all but three were based on fewer than one hundred cases. These three found a significant increase in risk for current estrogen users.[35] The Nurses' Study researchers concluded, "These data together with other epidemiological data and laboratory evidence suggest that estrogen is a promoter of mammary tumors," and that "the addition of progesterone [progestin] to estrogen therapy does not remove the elevation in risk."[36]

Other recent studies have reached similar results. A review of prior studies published in *Obstetrics and Gynecology* in February of 1992 found a 63 percent increase in breast cancer risk for women currently on HRT.[37] A Canadian study reported in 1992, involving 699 women with breast cancer and matched controls, confirmed that current estrogen users were 40 percent more likely to contract breast cancer than never-users. Unlike the Nurses' Study, however, it found that long-term hormone users were at even greater risk—60 percent more than never-users.[38] The 1989 Swedish study concurred, finding a 50 percent greater risk for estrogen use of nine years or more.[39]

The message seems to be that women should not take these powerful substances indefinitely. The problem is, when you discontinue the drugs you also lose their benefits. As soon as you stop taking estrogen, its cardiovascular benefits cease.[40] Rapid bone loss also occurs.[41] To forestall bone loss, you may need to take estrogen for life. The trade-off could be hip fractures for breast cancer, and even then it may not save your bones.[42] Again, there are safer and more effective alternatives.

The Nurses' Study researchers called the increase in risk a "modest" one. However, as Bruce Ettinger, M.D., Professor of Medicine and Radiology at the University of California, San Francisco, points out, "in terms of epidemiologic studies, a relative risk of 1.3 or 1.4 is small," but "in terms of an individual woman's concern, a 30 percent or 40 percent increase in breast cancer risk is large, especially since a woman's average lifetime risk of developing breast cancer is one in nine."[43]

For women whose symptoms are due to a true estrogen shortage, supplemental estrogen in the amount actually needed by the body should do no harm. The problem is in the wholesale prescription of ERT or HRT to all postmenopausal women, on the theory that if they don't need it for symptoms, they need it to prevent heart disease and osteoporosis.

Estrogen increases the risk not only of breast cancer but of uterine cancer. Both are particularly threatening to women in the menopausal years. The attempt to avoid cancer of the uterus is a leading reason why twenty-five percent of American women now reach menopause prematurely and abruptly by way of hysterectomy.[44]

Hysterectomy is one of several cancer prevention procedures that are now being questioned. Before we get to the natural alternatives, let's take a look at current cancer prevention techniques. Can we rely on them to allay breast and uterine cancer risks? Recent research is disquieting.

Chapter Five

Primary Prevention:
Menopause by Surgery and Drugs

Hysterectomy is one of the few major operations done by the gynaecologist and pride, technical practice, and financial incentive may generate a bias toward [it].
> —Dr. Lorraine Dennerstein,
> University of Melbourne[1]

The ultimate solution to the threat of uterine cancer is hysterectomy—surgical removal of the uterus. After all, we've been told, our female organs are of no further use after we've had our allotted number of children. We might as well have these organs removed to avoid future dangers of cancer and unwanted pregnancies. The ovaries are often removed as well. The ovaries produce estrogen, and estrogen stimulates uterine cancers to grow.

Hysterectomy has seen a dramatic increase in recent years. It is now one of the most performed surgical procedures in the United States, where the hysterectomy rate is *six times* that in Europe. One of every four American women reaching menopause does so artificially in the operating room.

Hysterectomy, however, is another solution with problems. For the nearly three quarters of a million American women who embark on menopause prematurely by surgery, the abruptness of the change wreaks havoc on hormone balance. It can bring on severe hot flashes within twenty-four hours of the operation. To counter these, most women resort to lifelong estrogen replacement. Many of these women are still young. In less than a decade, from 1965 to 1973, surgical removal of the uterus and ovaries nearly doubled in women 25 to 34 years old.[2]

Hysterectomy can also result in the prolapse of other organs, including the intestines, bowels, bladder, and vagina, causing pelvic pain, sexual problems, or pressure on the bowels and bladder. There can be other long-term complications as well, including osteoporosis, bone and joint pain, immobility, chronic fatigue, urinary problems, emotional problems, depression, and increased risk of heart disease. The Nurses' Health Study found that for women who have both ovaries removed and are not on hormone replacement therapy, the risk of a nonfatal heart attack is twice that of other women.[3] Unfortunately, at present a quarter of all women undergoing hysterectomies before age forty have both ovaries removed.[4] And even when they don't, in more than a third of cases the ovaries simply die following hysterectomy, and menopause follows.[5]

A less obvious problem involves sexual response. Debbie found this out to her dismay. Before her hysterectomy, sex for Debbie was very important. It gave her a zest for life and a kind of erotic excitement for everything she did. She liked feeling sexy and desirable, and considered it an integral part of who she was. Thus when her gynecologist said she needed to have her uterus removed to correct a uterine prolapse, she questioned him heavily before she consented to the procedure. Would it change her sexual desire and sensation? Would it lead to vaginal dryness? He assured her that nothing would change.

In fact, her sex life changed drastically. She not only experienced vaginal dryness but lost all sexual desire and the zest for life that went with it. When she told these complaints to her doctor, he said other women didn't experience them. He referred her to a psychiatrist.

Debbie is now extremely depressed, and angry at her doctor. She is suing him for misrepresentation, but the procedure is lengthy and unpromising. He can fall back on the pronouncement of a 1947 study that has formed prevailing American theory ever since:

Not only does this study deny the idea that the cervix is a necessary organ to be stimulated in order to achieve orgasm, but it also shows that neither uterus nor ovaries are necessary for its attainment.... Where there are changes in libido or sexual satisfaction following hysterectomy, the cause of these changes is undoubtedly psychogenic.[6]

It wasn't until the eighties that this idea was examined and found wanting. British researchers observed that in recent studies in the United Kingdom, 33 to 46 percent of women reported decreased sexual response after hysterectomy or oophorectomy (removal of the uterus and ovaries).[7]

In normal women, the ovaries continue to secrete some hormones for many years after menopause.[8] One hormone they continue to secrete is the androgen testosterone, which encourages libido. It causes increased susceptibility to sexual stimulation, increased sensitivity, and greater intensity of sexual gratification. Replacing estrogen with HRT doesn't replace this lost libido-stimulating hormone. Estrogen can encourage sexual response by counteracting genital dryness, atrophy and hot flashes; but studies show it does not actually restore libido.[9] (Supplementing with natural progesterone, on the other hand, can have this restorative effect, as we'll see later.)

For some women, the cervix and uterus are important for another reason: they are major triggers for orgasm.[10] As one hysterectomized woman was quoted in a clinical study:

> Before, each time the penis [was] pushed hard against the cervix, I would feel intense excitement deep inside me, huge waves of pleasure going from the area of the cervix all through my torso. This was by far the most exciting part of sex for me, the real climax. I've tried to be satisfied with the orgasms I get from stimulation of the clitoris, that is, mildly pleasurable contractions in the muscles in the front part of the vagina. Maybe I'll get used to it in time, but it isn't nearly as good, and I feel very sad.[11]

The loss of testosterone that comes with hysterectomy can be corrected with the implantation of testosterone pellets; but there's not much that can be done for the loss of sexual contractions of the cervix and uterus, except avoiding the surgery.

We'll look at alternatives to hysterectomy in Chapter Twelve. What we want to stress here is that it's not a procedure to be rushed into lightly, and neither is a hormone replacement therapy that increases its likelihood.

Fibroid tumors are the most common tumors of the female pelvic organs and the most frequent reason given for hysterectomy. They are rarely malignant, but they can cause excessive menstrual bleeding and pelvic pain that precipitates hysterectomy. Estrogen stimulates their growth. If estrogen levels are allowed to drop off naturally after menopause, existing uterine tumors will typically atrophy away by themselves; but when the hormone is artificially supplied, uterine tumors are stimulated to grow. Hysterectomy may be the result.[12]

Primary prevention for breast cancer: Menopause by drugs

"Primary prevention" is prevention that catches the disease before it starts. If primary prevention for uterine cancer is hysterectomy, the logical corrollary for breast cancer is mastectomy (removal of the breast). Some high-risk women have actually agreed to this mutilating surgery before they contracted the disease, but few women are willing to go to such drastic lengths.

Breast cancer, like endometrial cancer, is estrogen-dependent. Estrogen stimulates it to grow. Another surgical option that has been tried in the past is the removal of the organs that produce estrogen— the ovaries, the adrenals, and even the pituitary. Now, however, it is more common to suppress estrogen production with anti-estrogen drugs.

Currently, the best hope for primary prevention of breast cancer is considered to be the anti-cancer drug tamoxifen (Nolvadex, made by ICI Americas, Inc.).[13] The drug is being tested in a large-scale clinical trial sponsored by the U.S. National Cancer Institute (NCI) and the National Institutes of Health, in which women without symptoms are being given it and then watched for developments.

Volunteers have rushed to be included in the five-year, $60 million NCI study. Four thousand women—one-fourth of the 16,000 sought—called the NCI's telephone hotline within three days of the study's announcement in the spring of 1992. Many women felt the government was finally responding to claims that research into women's health has been sorely neglected.

The rush to volunteer reflected women's serious concerns about breast cancer risk. The hope that tamoxifen will reduce it is based on studies in which the drug has reduced cancer occurrence in the second breast of women who already had it in one breast. The problem is, the finding may have no relevance for healthy women without breast cancer.[14]

The tamoxifen study also raises ethical questions. It is the first major government study in which a substance known to have serious side effects and risks has been given to healthy people just to see if it might prevent disease later. The more likely outcome, according to Adrian Fugh-Berman, M.D., writing in *The Nation* in December of 1992, is that these women will develop diseases they wouldn't have been subject to otherwise.

Dr. Fugh-Berman says that researchers postulate the study will result in sixty-two prevented cases of breast cancer. In exchange for that benefit, 7,938 women receiving the drug will be subjected to risks and side effects without benefits to themselves. Tamoxifen users face a 500 percent increase in the risk of cancer of the endometrium, blood clots that can be fatal, eye damage, hepatitis and liver failure. The drug also causes liver cancer in rats. And since tamoxifen works by suppressing estrogen, its most common side effects are menopausal symptoms: hot flashes, vaginal discharge or dryness, irregular menstruation, depression and insomnia.[15]

"In recent years," commented Dr. Fugh-Berman, "the medical profession has tended more and more to accord risk factors—such as hypertension and high cholesterol—the status of diseases, for which the inherent risks and side effects of medical treatment are consequently acceptable. This mindset has generated a new category of patient: people who have nothing wrong with them but a statistical possibility. Such 'patients' become trapped in the endless medical maze of office visits, lab tests and drug therapy."

She added, "That the NCI has undertaken the tamoxifen study is all the more curious and disturbing in view of the fact that it has repeatedly rejected proposals to investigate possible links between a high-fat diet and breast cancer, and the possible preventive effects of a diet extremely low in fat." Dietary trials would not have exposed volunteers to side effects. Why did the NCI choose instead to study a drug? One suspects that the push from drug companies to sell their products, or to get government funding for FDA new-use studies, was a compelling factor. The NCI's ties with big business are notorious.[16] The cheapest way to finance studies complying with the FDA's stringent requirements is to persuade the government to underwrite the cost.

More disturbing than the potential misuse of government funds is the fact that women are recruited who may be ignorant of the risks they are running. Dr. Fugh-Berman concludes of the tamoxifen trial, "In place of the public health principle of great benefit for tiny risk, the Breast Cancer Prevention Trial offers a different and dangerous model: the substitution of one disease for another."[17]

So much for primary prevention. What about "secondary prevention," the Early Detection that is supposed to catch cancer at an easily-treated initial stage?

Chapter Six

Early Detection: "Prevention"
That Can Spread The Disease

Cancer diagnosis is a huge medical business, fanned by the public's fear of the disease and forty years of publicity by the American Cancer Society.
—Ralph W. Moss, Ph.D., former assistant director of public affairs at Memorial Sloan-Kettering Cancer Center[1]

"Never fear," said Dorothy's gynecologist when he put her on HRT. "Breast cancer risk can be allayed by early detection." But as her breasts were yanked into position and subjected to the Big Squeeze that made them red and sore for hours afterwards, she wondered if there wasn't a better way.

Even the National Cancer Institute is starting to wonder. Until recently it recommended mammograms, or x-rays of the breast, every year or two for all women over forty; but it has had to re-examine its position in the light of recent evidence. On June 2, 1991, the *London Times* published an article titled "Breast Scans Boost Risk of Cancer Death." Its opening line: *"Middle-aged women who have regular mammograms are more likely to die from breast cancer than women who are not screened, according to dramatic new research."*

The study reported the results of the Canadian National Breast Screening Study (NBSS), the largest study of its kind carried out anywhere in the world. The NBSS tracked 89,835 Canadian women aged forty to forty-nine during the period 1980–88. Half were given mammograms every twelve to eighteen months. The other half were given only a single physical exam.

To the surprise and chagrin of the researchers, at the end of the eight-year period, deaths among the group getting regular mammograms were "significantly higher" than in the group getting none. How much higher no one would say. The researchers said the results would be published later that year, but 1991 passed without the promised report.

In June of 1992, however, the NCI acknowledged that the increase in breast cancer deaths was a full 52 percent.[2] In other words, you were half again as likely to die of breast cancer if you *did* get regular mammograms as if you *didn't*.

This was alarming news to the cancer industry, which has been trying to explain it away ever since. The NCI reported that the director of the study, Professor Anthony Miller of the National Cancer Institute of Toronto, had retracted his warnings, since "mortality in the control group of 40 to 49 year olds is catching up." But when the study was finally published in November of 1992, the odds of dying of breast cancer if you had been screened were still reported to be 36 percent greater than if you had not.[3]

Miller's "retraction" (he himself denies making it) looks suspiciously political. The NCI noted that his original figures "*escaped* to the press" (the researchers would have preferred to keep them quiet); and Miller defended himself to his colleagues by saying, "The problem is that none of this was generated by us. In the context of trying to avoid anxiety for people and major problems for women, we have been saying more than possibly is appropriate.... But given the public health implications, we had no option."[4]

Miller maintains that the mammography was adequate and that the machines and radiation dosages were intensely monitored, so the excess deaths can't be blamed on unsafe levels of radiation. Then what caused the deaths? He suggested that cancer cells may have been squeezed into the bloodstream under the pressure of the mammographic plates. Alternatively, the excess deaths may have been in women who harbored a gene that increased the risk of radiation-induced breast cancer.

But these theories, too, may have been political afterthoughts. In the original *London Times* report, Miller asserted there was no evidence to suggest that the excess deaths were caused by the mammograms themselves. Rather, he thought, *the failures were in the cancer treatment that followed the diagnoses*.

"Studies in animals suggested that removal of the main tumour and radiation of the immediate area affected the body's immune system so that tumours elsewhere grow faster," he said. "Therefore one potential problem was that surgery, the anaesthetic and radiotherapy involved in treating women with breast cancer were interfering with immunity." As a result, "the initial radiation and surgery to remove tiny breast lumps discovered by mammograms may make secondary cancers elsewhere grow faster."

"You may find the cancers earlier (with mammography), but the women are still going to die," Miller said. "Modern treatment does not work for these early cancers."

The problem is, it was the *early* cancers that the cancer establishment had been telling us modern treatment does work for. The late cancers, the ones that had spread to other areas of the body, were known to be much harder to cure. It was to catch the early cancers that billions have been spent on mass screening for early detection.

A second look at early detection

The theory behind early detection to find impalpable cancers is that the earlier you catch them, the better your chances of survival. But as Petr Skrabanek observed in *The British Medical Journal* in 1985, "There is no evidence that early mastectomy affects survival. If the patients knew this, they would most likely refuse surgery."[5]

Dr. Hardin Jones, professor of medical physics and physiology at the University of California, Berkeley, extended this shocking statement to cancer treatment in general. "Serious attempts to relate prompt treatment with chance of cure have been unsuccessful," he told an American Cancer Society panel in 1969. He observed that subjects typically chosen for cancer treatments were patients considered operable and curable. Inoperable, terminal patients were left in the untreated control groups. After correcting for this bias, he said,

"My studies have proven conclusively that untreated cancer victims actually live up to four times longer than treated individuals."[6]

That was twenty-five years ago, but there is little information on the progress of untreated cancer that is more recent. Surgery became standard cancer treatment in the nineteenth century, long before controlled studies became popular. Today, nearly every cancer patient receives either surgery, radiation, or chemotherapy, so surveys of untreated patients are rare. Besides Dr. Jones' survey, another was conducted by Dr. H.J.G. Bloom, who wrote in the *British Journal of Cancer* in 1965:

> It is indeed a remarkable finding that patients who neglect the cancer in their breast for a year, or even longer, not infrequently appear to have a comparable or even better survival rate than do those women who seek advice after only a brief delay. This experience is not confined to breast cancer, and is also seen in reports concerning cancer of the stomach and rectum.[7]

If cancer treatment has improved in recent years, it is not reflected in the death rate. A 1993 editorial in the British medical journal *The Lancet* cynically observes:

> Some readers may be startled to learn that the overall mortality rate from carcinoma of the breast remains static. If one were to believe all the media hype, the triumphalism of the profession in the published research, and the almost weekly miracle breakthroughs trumpeted by the cancer charities, one might be surprised that women are dying at all from this cancer.[8]

The fact is, the cancer death rate continues to rise at an alarming rate. In 1900, cancer accounted for one in twenty-seven deaths. In the sixties, it accounted for one in six deaths. In 1988, it accounted for one in five.[9] Breast cancer incidence has increased 30 percent since the seventies, when mammography came into vogue. Disturbing new research suggests a cause and effect relationship.

Early detection and the breast cancer epidemic

New studies suggest that the surge in breast cancer cases has resulted because mammography and biopsy are detecting "pre-cancerous" conditions that would not otherwise have turned into active cancers. That would make both the apparent incidence and the apparent cure rate go up, since the easiest cancers to cure are the ones that aren't really cancer. The disturbing part is that 30 percent of breast cancer "victims" may have been victims only of their unnecessary treatments: biopsy, surgery, radiation, and chemotherapy.

Breast cancer now takes one or both breasts of 150,000 women a year.[10] Even the National Cancer Institute now concedes that mass screening may be responsible for the statistical increase (or apparent increase) in breast cancer incidence.[11] The suspicion was strengthened by a recent study at Fred Hutchinson Cancer Research Center in Seattle. It found that the apparent increase in breast cancer could be explained by early detection alone.[12]

"If 'early' [detection] means premalignant lesions, then it could be too early," observed Dr. Skrabanek in 1985. "Evidence must be provided that such lesions would develop into an invasive cancer within the life-span of the bearer, if a potentially large number of unnecessary mastectomies is to be prevented."[13] Mastectomies are being replaced by lumpectomies that cut out less of the breast, but it's still a procedure you don't want to go through if you don't have to.

Some experts feel that the diagnostic biopsy that follows a suspicious mammogram can be even more dangerous than the surgery. Surgery involves cutting around the tumor in an attempt to "get it all." Biopsy, on the other hand, involves cutting *through* the protective shell that keeps the tumor from spreading. The incision itself can turn an inactive, encapsulated cancer into one that can metastasize (spread through the bloodstream). It's when cancer metastasizes that it becomes fatal.

"Even needle biopsy does not appear to be safe," noted Dr. George Crile Jr., Emeritus Surgeon of the Cleveland Clinic. "It gives credence to what our patients already think and tell us—that cutting into cancer spreads it and makes it grow."[14]

A German study that looked at the effects on survival of biopsies and needle biopsies for breast cancer found that biopsied patients died earlier than women whose malignancies were established by other means.[15] For most patients, biopsy risks are borne unnecessarily, since some eight or nine out of every ten biopsies done on the basis of a positive breast x-ray are negative.[16] In one series, nineteen out of twenty tumors that were biopsied were benign.[17]

Even if your biopsy turns out to be negative, it's not going to be good for your stress level. "For a woman who has been told that she may have breast cancer," says Dr. J. E. Devitt of the University of Ottawa, "the anguish is the same whether or not she has a tumour. This worry starts with the first suggestion that she may have the disorder and lasts until a final decision of innocence is made—usually a few weeks but possibly some months later. For every woman with breast cancer, there will be six healthy women who will also have to endure the anxiety associated with that diagnosis.... The anxiety due to these false alarms can only be appreciated by those who have endured it."[18]

Dr. Devitt reported the results of a survey of 2,923 women seen for breast problems in a consulting surgical practice from 1985 through 1988. Of 237 mammograms suggesting cancer, 220—or 93 percent—turned out to be false alarms. Eighty-six percent of cancer signs and symptoms detected by routine physical examination, and 88 percent of those detected by breast self-examination, also proved to be false alarms.

Dr. Devitt maintains that about half of these anguishing false positives could be eliminated by proper education, and by delaying breast examination until certain ages. In his series, 30 percent of false positives could have been avoided by educating patients to understand that unless a lump is obvious, breast pain and nipple discharge are not usually symptoms of breast cancer. Another 20 percent could have been avoided by postponing routine physical examination to the age of forty-five, postponing breast self-examination to the age of thirty-five, and postponing mammography to the age of sixty.[19]

The latter suggestion was supported by Part II of the Canadian National Breast Screening Study, involving women aged fifty to fifty-nine. In this age group the value of mammography was thought to be firmly established. However, the researchers found that no fewer deaths from breast cancer resulted in women getting mammograms in their fifties than in those not getting them.[20]

These findings suggest that for women in general, the current demand for more and cheaper screening may be misguided. But for women on estrogen, the delay in screening recommended by Dr. Devitt could be risky since their increased breast cancer risk mandates regular monitoring.

Secondary prevention for uterine cancer

If you take estrogen, not only your breasts but your uterus and cervix will be monitored for cancer. Most doctors do an endometrial biopsy before starting a woman on hormone replacement, and another biopsy or a Pap smear to monitor developments within the next six months. A Pap smear is likely to be required every six months thereafter. An aspiration biopsy will then be required whenever there is any indication of abnormal endometrial buildup, including any irregular bleeding. Physicians are required by law to do a biopsy or ultrasound of the uterine lining whenever a patient bleeds midcycle. This bleeding, unfortunately, is common in women on HRT.[21]

Biopsies are a form of surgery, and are painful and disturbing to patients. However, the less invasive Pap smear isn't sufficient for detecting uterine cancer, because you can't rely on it to pick up abnormal tissue in the uterus. Pap smears are designed only for cervical examination.[22]

Even as a test for cervical cancer, some experts question the Pap smear's worth. Dr. James McCormick of Trinity College, Dublin, notes that the test is highly unreliable, producing both false positives and false negatives; and there are no randomized controlled trials showing it actually saves lives. The closest attempt was a trial in Canada, where mass cervical screening was done in British Columbia but not in the rest of the country. Deaths from cervical cancer did drop in British Columbia, but they also dropped in the rest of the country, and to the same extent.[23]

In the United Kingdom, on the other hand, the death rate has not dropped despite 40 million smears. Ironically, deaths from cervical cancer were rare to start with. Notes Dr. McCormick, "a general practitioner would not be expected to sign a death certificate with this diagnosis more than once or twice in a professional lifetime." A 1990 American study reported that the cost of allowing one person to live one year longer by annual Pap tests is $930,000.[24]

In the U.S., like the U.K., the Pap smear is not only one of the most common and popular laboratory tests but one of the most unreliable. In one study, experts disagreed on whether cancer cells were present in about 40 percent of the cervical smears examined. In another study, in about two-thirds of the cases studied, two Pap smears taken at the same time from the same woman showed different results.[25]

Despite these provisos, we are *not* saying you should avoid diagnostic tests. What we want to suggest is that you should think twice about exposing yourself to known cancer promoters like estrogen and then relying on early detection to ward off cancer. Early detection is not prevention. Once cancer has been detected, you've already got the disease; and both the diagnosis and the treatment can actually compound your risks.

II

Natural Hormones

The Chinese believe that the original insult to each meridian or energy system is emotional, and that each emotion disturbs a different meridian. For the liver meridian, it's anger. For the kidney meridian, it's fear. The kidney meridian is the energy system governing reproductive function, including conception, growth, and development.

Anger and fear are emotions characteristic of the stressful lives of many people, both men and women. Suppressed, built-up anger causes the liver energy to stagnate. Stagnation is one way excess energy is drawn to the liver meridian from the kidney meridian. When the kidney meridian is weakened, an early menopause and menopausal symptoms can result.

Menopause itself (the cessation of monthly periods) is treated by Oriental doctors as a natural occurrence resulting in less blood production. The process of regularly producing enough blood to nourish a fetus places a burden on the kidney (the energy system governing reproductive function). If allowed to continue indefinitely, this process would prematurely exhaust the kidneys and lead to early aging and debility. So the body shifts into a new mode, in which its *Qi* or life force is no longer sent down from the heart to the uterus through the blood to produce a new physical life but is sent up to the heart to nourish the woman's spirit. This *Qi* reversal allows the postmenopausal woman to become the wise woman or *sage femme*, the mother of her community and a fountain of wisdom. For Chinese women, menopause is looked forward to for its potential for gaining wisdom and spiritual power.[2]

Chinese herbs

Imbalances in the system are corrected by Chinese doctors with traditional herbal formulas whose safety and effectiveness have been proven through centuries of use. Publications from the People's Republic of China report that Chinese herbal formulas are effective in a broad range of clinical situations.[3] Balance is also achieved with acupuncture, a technique that involves placing very fine needles in specific locations to facilitate the flow of *Qi* throughout the body.

The Chinese consider menopause to be a deficiency of blood and Yin (the fluids of the body). Treatment is with natural remedies that strengthen and build the blood. One advantage of this approach is that you don't have to take the remedies forever. You need them only until your Yin is built back up and your body is back in balance. However, you may want to continue to take different Chinese herbs as your body's needs change.

Dr. Walker has seen Chinese herbal formulas resolve menopausal and premenstrual symptoms ranging from the common to the bizarre. Sylvia's chief complaint was in the latter category. Her tongue, she said, was burning hot. Her doctor told her she would just have to live with it, but Sylvia said she couldn't. Dr. Walker gave her a Chinese remedy for the symptom complex known in Chinese medical terminology as "heart-fire." Sylvia's menopausal problems disappeared. "I'm thrilled," Sylvia beamed. "The doctor told me I had to live with it, and I don't."

Marlene complained of continual hot flashes, irritability, and a desire to jump out of her skin. Her tongue was red and dry, indicating a Yin deficiency. Her symptoms were relieved by a Chinese formula called *Quiet Contemplative*. "I feel like a new woman," she said after using this single remedy. "I feel twenty years younger."

Phil came into Capitol Drugs looking for a remedy for his wife. He said she suffered from vaginal dryness so severe that their sex life was virtually non-existent. Dr. Walker suggested the classic Chinese formula *Women's Journey*. Phil was smiling broadly when he came back to confirm that the remedy had worked.

Mary, age forty-four, is a high-powered business woman under a great deal of stress. Recently, she had been so agitated and distracted that she had little patience with her employees. She suffered from spontaneous sweating, irritability, and hot flashes. Her tongue was red with a purple cast, indicating a stagnation of liver energy. Dr. Walker gave her the two principal Chinese formulas for menopause, *Relaxed Wanderer* followed by *Quiet Contemplative*. Her symptoms, too, went away, to the relief of both Mary and her co-workers.

Relaxed Wanderer, the brand name for a Chinese patent formula called *Hsaio Yao Wan* (or *Xiao Yao Tang*), is an excellent remedy not only for menopausal complaints but for PMS. Dr. Walker has recommended it to several hundred PMS patients, and the vast majority have reported being delighted with the results. The remedy works in widespread use from 1947 to 1964. It was discontinued at that time only after large numbers of female children born to mothers on the drug were found to have a higher risk of vaginal cancer.

Unopposed Premarin continued to be popular for menopausal complaints until 1975, when an astute cancer statistician in San Francisco noticed that uterine cancer in the Bay Area had risen by fifty percent since 1969, and had doubled among women over fifty in wealthy Marin County. The epidemic was traced to oral estrogen, prescriptions for which had also tripled between 1965 and 1975.[4] Later studies showed that unopposed estrogen increases the risk of endometrial cancer (cancer of the lining of the uterus) by 400 to 800 percent.[5] The increased risk does not stop when a woman stops taking the drug but continues for many years afterwards.[6]

This alarming result was soon explained as a problem of imbalance. Estrogen was being supplied without its antagonist progesterone. In a normal menstrual cycle, estrogen is released in the first part of the cycle and builds up the lining of the endometrium. After ovulation, midway through the cycle, progesterone is released to prepare the lining of the uterus to nurture a fertilized egg. If no egg attaches, progesterone production stops and menstruation starts. The endometrial buildup stimulated by estrogen is then sloughed off and eliminated. The problem with ERT was that it artificially replaced only one of the hormones lost at menopause. Without progesterone, the uterine lining could continue to build up, producing the uncontrolled proliferation of cells known as cancer.

The logical correction for this imbalance was to add progesterone to the formula. It would check the proliferation of endometrial cells and thus reduce the risk of endometrial cancer. Although some gynecologists still prescribe estrogen alone, the prevailing trend in the U.S. since the mid-seventies has been toward the estrogen/progesterone mixture, collectively called HRT or Hormone Replacement Therapy.

The "progesterone" used in HRT is actually a synthetic product. Synthetic "progestins" or "progestogens" are substances having progesterone-like effects. (For simplicity, we'll use the term "progestins" here for both.) Provera (medroxyprogesterone acetate) is the most popular brand for use in HRT. Other commonly used progestins are Amen, Norlutin, and Norlutate. Protection against uterine cancer seems to require their use for two weeks at the end of each 25-day course of estrogen.

Adding a progestin to the formula solved the problem of endometrial cancer, but brought other problems. Progestins are not real progesterone. To date no synthetic progestin has been able to duplicate the hormonal activities of the native hormone.[7]

Keeping up HRT

Gail Sheehy described her problems with Provera in her book *Silent Passage*. "After only a month," she wrote, "the estrogen had rekindled sexual desire, stopped the surges of static and dips of fatigue, and chased away the blues. But the Provera was another matter. It brought on unbelievable physical and emotional symptoms that I'd never experienced before. After a year of the combined hormones, my body seemed to be at war with itself for half of every month. My energy was flagging, and resistance to minor infections was falling. I felt as if I were racing my motor. So I stopped taking hormones cold turkey."[8]

The problem with Provera and other chemically altered forms of progesterone is that they are not as good a "fit" as the natural hormone. They perform some but not all of its functions. They cannot, like natural progesterone, be converted in the body to other hormones as needed. They also come with a host of side effects, including bloating, water retention, nausea, insomnia, jaundice, mental depression, fever, masculinization, weight changes, breast tenderness, abdominal cramping, anxiety, irritability, and allergic reactions. Fluid retention can exacerbate asthma, migraines, epilepsy, and heart and kidney problems.[9]

Although these compounds are allowed to go under the name of progesterone, some are actually two thousand times more potent than the form found in the body. Some are made strictly from chemicals. Others are made from the male hormone testosterone. Androgenic (male-type) progestins, including norethynodrel, ethisterone, dimesthisterone and norethisterone (used in birth control pills), react like male hormones and can give you masculine characteristics. Oth-

Chapter Seven

Herbs East and West

O! mickle is the powerful grace that lies
In herbs, plants, stones, and their true qualities.
                                        —*Romeo and Juliet*

The problem with recommending estrogen for all menopausal women is that many women are already in a state of estrogen dominance. Adding more of the hormone can encourage cancer growth. A safer approach would be to supply the body with whatever it needs to balance its own hormones, producing more or less as required. The ideal remedy for menopausal and premenstrual complaints would be one that eliminates symptoms without short-term or long-term side effects, and without increasing cancer risk. Oriental and Western herbal formulas, homeopathic remedies, and natural plant-based progesterone are all candidates.

Lynne Walker recommends natural remedies to patients in her private practice as an acupuncturist and homeopath and as a consultant at Capitol Drugs, a holistic drugstore in Sherman Oaks, California. There she advises many patients a day and has very little time with each one. She has been successful in solving their menopausal and premenstrual complaints, by recommending one or two of the popular Chinese or American herbal formulas or homeopathic remedies designed for particular symptom complexes. The remedies, she says, are easy to select and they work. They are just not well known.

In this chapter, we'll look at Oriental and Western herbal remedies. In the next chapter, we'll look at homeopathy.

The Oriental approach

From the point of view of Oriental medicine, supplementing the body's own estrogen and progesterone are stopgap measures. Chinese remedies rebalance the body so that it can produce its own hormones, tapering off gradually and imperceptibly as the material function of giving birth is replaced with the more spiritual interests of old age.

Chinese doctors see health as a state of harmonious balance of the body's *Qi* energy or vital life force. Disruption of the flow of the vital force to any organ causes an imbalance throughout the system. The more out of balance the system is, the more likely that PMS, menopausal symptoms, and midlife cancers will result.

According to Chinese medical theory, *Qi* flows in set patterns throughout the energy systems of the body. These energy patterns are called meridians and are named for the major organs they pass through (heart, stomach, lung, kidney, liver). The energy flows through them in a circular pattern as illustrated in Figure 2.[1]

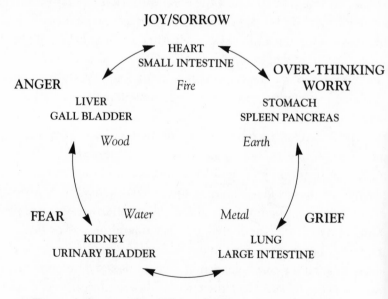

Figure 2. Energy Flow Through Major Organ Systems

particularly well for women with a tendency to be cold (e.g., to have cold hands and feet). For women who are perimenopausal and tend to be hot, *Bupleurum and Peony Formula* is likely to be more effective.

For menopausal complaints including restlessness and hot flashes, acupuncturist Janet Zand favors the Chinese patent formula *Zhi Bai Di Huang Tang.* Her company's version is called *Anem-Phello and Rehmannia Formula.* The K'an Herb version is called *Temper Fire.*

The Chinese patent and American brand names of some popular Chinese formulas for women's complaints are listed in Figure 3. In this and the following charts of products, we've included brand names and manufacturers, but we don't mean to limit your choice to particular brands. These are products currently popular at Capitol Drugs, where Dr. Walker is familiar with customer demand.

The components of the traditional Chinese formulas include hormones derived from plants. Plant estrogens are much weaker than prescription estrogens and are more easily absorbed and used by the body. They are quite effective, yet they avoid the strong side effects of prescription estrogen.

Dong quai or Tang-Kwei (*Angelica sinensis* root), is a highly effective remedy for hot flashes although its estrogen content is only 1/400th that of drugstore estrogen. Clinical and laboratory studies have shown *Dong quai* to be effective in stimulating uterine contractions; resolving blood clots; increasing the metabolism of the body and the oxygen consumption of the liver; lowering blood pressure; protecting the cardiovascular system; fighting bacteria and viruses; and reducing water retention.[4] When used in combination with other herbs, *Dong quai* is an effective antidote for menopausal anxiety, depression, nervousness and insomnia. Results may take a week or two, but homeopathic remedies can be used in the meantime for relief of symptoms (see Chapter Eight).

Another common Chinese herbal component is *Ginseng.* The two main species of this plant are the Chinese or Oriental (*Panax ginseng*) and American (*Panax quinquefolium*) forms. Considered the king of all medicinal herbs, in China *ginseng* is the most extensively used Chi-strengthening medicine. Clinical and laboratory studies have shown that it stimulates, regulates, and normalizes the central nervous system; stimulates and strengthens the heart; normalizes the blood pressure; regulates blood sugar; stimulates and regulates the pituitary, thyroid, and adrenal glands; combats stress and shock; and enhances the body's resistance to cancer.[5] In menopausal women, it naturally stimulates estrogen production without risk.

Chinese name	U.S. formulation	Made by*
Hsiao Yao Wan (Xiao Yao Tang)	Relaxed Wanderer	K'an Herbs
	Bupleurum & Peony Formula	McZand
Liu Wei Di Huang Wan	Quiet Contemplative	K'an Herbs
	Rehmannia Six Formula	McZand
Zhi Bhi Ba Wei Wan (Eight Flavored Tea)	Rehmannia 8	Chinese Traditional Formulas
Wen Jing Tang	Women's Journey	K'an Herbs
Tang Kuei	Tang Kuei	Jade
	Bupleurum & Tang Kuei Formula	McZand
Zhi Bai Di Huang Tang	Anem-Phello & Rehmannia Formula	McZand
	Temper Fire	K'an Herbs
		*See Appendix.

Figure 3. Chinese Herbs: Popular Patent Formulas for Menopause

Siberian ginseng (Eleutherococcus senticosus root) is not a true ginseng but is grouped with it because of similar active chemicals and physiological effects. It is used to increase longevity and decrease weakness and fatigue.

Bupleurum is used in Chinese herbal formulas to reduce liver inflammation and congestion. The liver is where female hormones are converted into usable compounds.

Peony (*Radix paeoniae lactiflorae*) is a Chinese herb that nourishes the blood. It is used for deficient blood patterns including menstrual dysfunction, leukorrhea (vaginal discharge), and uterine bleeding. It is also used for spontaneous sweating and night sweats, caused in Chinese medical terminology by deficient Yin that allows the fiery Yang to surface.[6]

These are just a few of the herbal components in the classical Chinese formulas, which contain herbs in traditional combinations that have been proven safe and effective over centuries. It's important to take Chinese herbs in the balanced formulas that address your whole symptom complex, since if you take them singly you run the risk of throwing your body further out of balance.

Western herbs

The European and native American Indian herbal traditions also include excellent botanicals for premenstrual and menopausal complaints.

One of these herbal remedies resolved Janet's mounting struggle with PMS. Half the month Janet was calm and pleasant, a joy to her husband and the employees at the restaurant she managed. But about a week before her period, she went out of control. She reacted with anger at small offenses that would have passed unnoticed the week before. Her husband suggested counseling, which she tried, but it didn't help. She visited a PMS clinic and was given synthetic progesterone in a rectal suppository form, but she had to quit taking it because it gave her diarrhea. She then consulted Dr. Walker, who gave her an American-made red raspberry leaf herbal combination formula. Amazingly, all her symptoms were relieved. Now, says Janet, she no longer feels she is losing control. She always "feels like herself."

Mindy was an acupuncture student with menstrual cramps so severe that she could not go to school on the day of her monthly period. Her problem was relieved by taking the same red raspberry leaf formula, beginning a week before her period.

Yvonne is a flight attendant who, at fifty, is just completing her education for a second career in architecture. She went through a bitter divorce and is still involved in a custody battle for her daughter. Yvonne is physically and emotionally stressed; yet a year ago she breezed through menopause without symptoms—no hot flashes, no mood swings, no fatigue. She simply stopped having menstrual periods. What was her secret? She isn't sure herself, but she does mention that about ten years ago she started taking certain herbal formulas whose ingredients included red raspberry and black cohosh. They were recommended by an iridologist to combat fatigue after her pregnancy. They gave her a lift, so she's been taking them ever since. Did these herbs keep her hormones in balance so that she never experienced the erratic surges experienced by other highly stressed women? It's not a controlled study, but it is an intriguing possibility.

Red raspberry leaf (*Rubus idaeus*) is one of the most popular Western herbs for correcting hormone imbalances. A member of the rose family, it is an example of the naturopathic principle that a remedy needn't be strong to be effective or wide-ranging in its effects. Red raspberry is best taken in the form of a simple infusion or tea. It restores and harmonizes uterine functions and helps rebuild uterine tissue, making it one of the few herbs that can actually be strongly recommended throughout pregnancy. It also arrests bleeding and discharge and is useful in the treatment of uterine prolapse and mild digestive complaints, including diarrhea and constipation.

Black cohosh (*Cimicifuga racemosa* or *black snake-root*) is an estrogen stimulant traditionally used for quelling hot flashes. In 1991, the mechanism for its observed benefits was confirmed in a controlled study. When 110 menopausal women were treated with extracts of the herb, their levels of luteinizing hormone (LH) declined. An elevation of LH has been linked to hot flashes.[7]

Another useful Western herb is chasteberry or monk's pepper (*Vitex agnus castus* root). It was a favorite in the Middle Ages but for other reasons: the peppery grey Mediterranean plant was valued by celibate monks for its ability to suppress sexual desire. Later research, however, revealed that it had this effect only in people afflicted with an excess of sexual desire. In "melancholic" people with the opposite affliction, it had the opposite effect. This balancing feature is chasteberry's strength for women's complaints. It works whether hormones are deficient or in excess, by stimulating the pituitary gland in the brain to harmonize hormone imbalances and make its own progesterone. The advantage of this option over supplemental hormones is that you cannot get too much. The herb will not force production of more than the body needs.

German research has shown that the chasteberry plant increases luteinizing hormone, which stimulates progesterone synthesis and secretion. It can also increase prolactin, which encourages milk production. Other studies have shown that the herb can regulate periods involving too frequent or too much bleeding. It's a good treatment for fibroids and for inflammation of the lining of the womb. However, it should not be used during pregnancy, since it's a strong uterine stimulant.[8]

Wild yam (*Dioscorea villosa*) contains a substance called diosgenin that can be converted in the laboratory to the human hormone progesterone. Wild yam has been used traditionally to treat inflammation, menstrual problems and (in small amounts) morning sickness.[9] Either Mexican wild yam (*Dioscorea barbasco*) or soybeans are the raw materials for the progesterone contained in the available natural progesterone and estrogen creams.

These are only a few of the more interesting Western herbs. Other popular varieties useful for correcting hormonal imbalances are listed in Figure 4.[10] Which extracts are right for your symptoms? You probably won't be able to tell from the labels, which the FDA requires to be vague; so again we recommend seeking the help of a competent naturopathic or homeopathic physician.

To locate an acupuncturist or naturopath in your area, you can try calling your State Board of Acupuncture or State Board of Naturopathy; but good practitioners are often unlisted, as are MDs who use holistic therapies. Another option is to ask around, get patient referrals, and choose a practitioner other women have been pleased with. You could also try calling a company that makes the products you're interested in and ask for a practitioner in your area who uses them. The fact that a practitioner uses particular products doesn't indicate competence; but you will at least have located one with some experience in their use. Manufacturers of natural products are listed in the Appendix.

To stimulate progesterone production:

Angelica sinensis	*Lady's mantle*	*White deadnettle*
Chasteberry	*Mugwort*	*Wild yam*
Elecampane	*Sarsaparilla*	*Yarrow*
Helonias	*Spikenard*	

To stimulate estrogen production:

Angelica archangelica	*Hops*	*Pomegranate husk*
Black cohosh	*Licorice*	*Sage*
Cypress	*Panax ginseng*	

To inhibit estrogen production:

Cumin	*Poppy*	*Stoneweed*
Pasque flower	*Rye ergot*	

To restore and tone the uterus:

Black haw	*Life root*	*White deadnettle*
Blue cohosh	*Red raspberry*	
Helonias	*Squaw vine*	

To treat uterine blood deficiency:

Angelica sinensis	*Helonias*	*Parsley root*
Artichoke	*Mugwort*	

To remineralize the bones:

Hemp nettle	*Knotweed*	*Stinging nettle*
Horsetail	*Lithothamnium calcareum (a seaweed)*	

For disturbances of the nervous system:

Black horehound	*Hawthorn berry*	*Lemon balm*

For diuresis and to counteract water retention:

Fennel	*Horse chestnut*	*Orthosiphon*
Grape vine leaf	*Meadowsweet*	*Witch hazel*

Combination formulas:

Female Formula (McZand)	Motherwort-Black Cohosh (Eclectic)
Menosan (Bioforce)	PMS Herbal (McZand)

Figure 4. Popular Botanicals Useful for Menopausal Complaints

Chapter Eight

Homeopathic Remedies

Through the like, disease is produced and through the application of the like it is cured.

—Hippocrates, fourth century B.C.

Other very effective treatments for menopausal complaints are homeopathic remedies. Originated in Germany, homeopathic medicine involves inducing a mild reaction in the body by simulating the larger reaction that constitutes the disease. Where "allopaths" (conventional doctors) suppress symptoms, homeopaths encourage them, on the theory that they represent the body's natural method of flushing toxins.

Homeopathic remedies consist of substances that, if given to healthy people in larger doses, would cause the symptoms the patient is experiencing. Side effects are avoided because the remedies are so diluted that no molecule of the original substance is likely to be left in solution.

These remedies work only if they have been "potentized" or energized through vigorous shaking, called "succussion." The succussion apparently transmits the energy pattern of the original substance to the neutral matter in which it was diluted (usually water and alcohol). Homeopaths say the effect of the remedies is electromagnetic rather than chemical, and that they act on the entire body at an energetic level. W. Ludwig, a modern German homeopath, observes that homeopathic medicines create a measurable effect in the stagnant circulation of patients' blood within seconds of intravenous injection, long before the medicine could have been physically distributed through the body in order to act chemically.[1]

In Europe, homeopathy has been widely accepted and practiced for two centuries. Today, according to the British Medical Journal, 32 percent of French family physicians and 20 percent of German physicians use it. In Great Britain, where its prestigious patrons include the Queen and Royal Family, 42 percent of physicians refer patients to homeopaths. These statistics are actually conservative, since Europeans brought up with homeopathy don't need a physician to prescribe remedies. Homeopathy is taught in medical school, so all physicians are "homeopathic physicians." Other countries in which homeopathy is popular include Australia, Canada, India, and most former English and French colonial countries in Africa. One indication of, and reason for its popularity in those countries is that homeopathy is covered by national health insurance.

In the United States, by contrast, acceptance of homeopathic medicine has been slower. Its fight for recognition has lasted for over a century.

Vicissitudes of an alternative medical approach

Although the homeopathic principle of "like cures like" goes back to Hippocrates, the concept was actually popularized by the German physician Samuel Hahnemann in the 1790s. In the great cholera epidemic of the 1830s, Hahnemann's remedies proved notably more effective than conventional treatment, and his fame spread. In the United States, homeopathy established medical societies and colleges in a growing number of states by the mid-nineteenth century. In 1844, the American Institute of Homeopathy was organized as the first national medical society.

Opposition mounted, however, when allopathic doctors saw homeopathy as a threat to their own market and counterattacked by forming the AMA. Its campaign was so effective that the 10,000 homeopaths and twenty homeopathic medical schools existing at the beginning of the twentieth century were reduced to less than 600 homeopaths and no exclusively homeopathic medical schools by the 1970s.[2]

Homeopathy's legal nadir may have been reached in 1990, when a North Carolina court revoked a physician's medical license for prescribing homeopathic medicines. There was nothing illegal about the remedies, which are available without a prescription. The doctor's crime was simply in using something no other M.D. was using in North Carolina. That meant he was not conforming to "prevailing medical practice," the standard of practice set forth in the medical practice act of North Carolina.[3]

Other states have similar medical practice acts, but few courts have construed them so strictly against homeopathy. The swing in many states seems to be in the other direction. Homeopathy is now accepted, recognized and regulated in Connecticut, Arizona, and Nevada; while new laws in Alabama and Washington State will make it easier for doctors to add it to their practices.[4]

Even allopathic drug companies are now developing homeopathic product lines. Fleet, which markets disposable enemas and douches, just came out with a homeopathic vaginal suppository. Homeopathy is gaining validity in the market largely because it is popular with consumers. Homeopathy is part of a recent medical self-care movement in America, which has as its goal empowering people to heal themselves knowledgeably without reliance on doctors.

Another reason for homeopathy's recent popularity is that a series of studies has finally brought scientific credence to the theory. While two centuries of empirical testing convinced families in the homeopathic tradition, conventional medicine had written it off because it involved doses so small that chemically they could have no effect. As late as 1988, for example, the FDA removed a homeopathic diet aid called "Appetoff" from the market, although research showed that 91.6 percent of people using it for at least one week lost weight. Despite proof of efficacy, the FDA concluded that the product must be fraudulent because no active ingredients could be detected in it.[5]

In June of 1988, however, the respected British publication *Nature* published a puzzling but dramatic study. It involved a special type of white blood cell which, when exposed to a particular antibody, is known to change chemically and structurally in a detectable way. In the experiment, these anticipated chemical and structural changes did occur. Yet the antibody had been diluted to 1 part per 10 to the 120th parts of distilled water—so dilute that no molecule of the original active ingredient was likely to be left. The results were so foreign to conventional theory that the editors themselves felt compelled to say they didn't believe them—although the study was performed by reputable researchers in six different laboratories at four major universities, in France, Israel, Italy and Canada—and was repeated *seventy* times.[6]

This was only one in a wave of well-designed studies supporting homeopathic theory. In recent years, nearly two dozen good double-blind studies have attested to the effectiveness of homeopathic remedies.[7]

A study testing homeopathic remedies for menopause and PMS was published in 1992. It involved the German remedy "Mulimen," composed of homeopathic doses of *Agnus castus* (chasteberry), *Cimicifuga racemosa* (black cohosh or black snake-root), *Hypericum* (St. John's wart), and *Sepia* (cuttlefish ink). Over a twelve-week period, 58 percent of 82 women treated with Mulimen for premenstrual and menopausal syndromes experienced significant relief of their symptoms. Although the study was not double-blind, half the women no longer experienced hot flashes, an objective result unlikely to be the product of suggestion.[8]

Homeopathic remedies for women's complaints

Homeopathic remedies can be surprisingly effective on menopausal and premenstrual symptoms. In the practice of Dr. Walker, a single, simple remedy has in many cases taken care of a patient's whole problem without side effects.

Natalie, age forty-four, said that three years ago she'd been treated for stomach problems after a trip to Colombia. Her doctor thought she was cured; but a few months later, her stomach was so irritated that she had to go back to him. This time he diagnosed ulcerative colitis and prescribed a sulfa drug called Azulfidine. He told her she would be on the drug for life. At first it seemed to help, but then Natalie entered "the Change." Physical changes at menopause can throw your body off so much that things that never bothered you before now become intolerable. Every time she took the drug, Natalie had an upset stomach, gas, and bloating. Her symptoms suggested intestinal parasites. Dr. Walker gave her a homeopathic remedy for parasites and told her what to expect: a huge diarrhea, followed by relief of her symptoms. Happily, that's just what happened.

Dolly, a forty-eight-year-old biker, came into Dr. Walker's office in tears. She complained of hot flashes, emotional ups and downs, and feelings of ambivalence. Dr. Walker recommended a combination product whose principal ingredient was *lachesis*, one of the most popular homeopathic remedies for menopausal symptoms. *Lachesis* contains homeopathic doses of the venom of a South American snake and has been used by homeopaths for nearly two centuries. When Dolly came back two days later and again two weeks later, she said the remedy had worked completely. She felt stable and rational again.

Another case of hot flashes was interesting because it involved a man. John, age fifty-two, complained of hot flashes after he'd been given a hormone-suppressing drug for prostate cancer. He too experienced immediate relief with *lachesis*, in combination with the Chinese herbal formula *Quiet Contemplative*.

Another effective product for hot flashes and night sweats recommended by homeopathic physician Fuller Royal, M.D., of the Nevada Clinic in Las Vegas, is a homeopathic version of the herb red raspberry leaf. It's a "gemmo therapy" product—a homeopathic remedy made from the plant's baby roots, which are believed to have more life force than other plant parts. The product is called *Rubus Idaeus* (the Latin name for the plant) and is manufactured by Dolisos.

To help preserve your bones, European homeopath and author Jan DeVries recommends a homeopathic product called *Urticalcin*, consisting of a combination of calcium and silica. It stabilizes the bones and prevents calcium loss by signalling the body to stop pulling calcium off the bones. In combination with evening primrose oil (discussed in Chapter Fifteen), it also helps provide the substrate necessary to manufacture better quality hormones.

Homeopathic remedies were grandfathered in under the 1962 amendments to the Food, Drug, and Cosmetic Act requiring extensive testing for effectiveness, so you can get them without a prescription. Unless you were brought up in a homeopathic family, how-ever, you may have trouble knowing which to use without profes-sional help. Your pharmacist is legally authorized to help you select among them, but most pharmacists know little about them. If you are choosing your own remedies, you need to either read up and become well-informed, or choose one of the prepared combination products that are more likely to be effective on a range of symptom complexes. Homeopathic remedies useful for menopausal and pre-menstrual complaints in particular cases, including some popular combination products, are listed in Figure 5.[9]

When choosing your own remedies, you should take only 3x to 30x potencies, nothing higher. Don't worry if your symptoms get worse before they get better; that's what they're supposed to do. This effect is called a "healing crisis" and shows that the remedy is encour-aging your body's toxin-flushing efforts. You should stop taking the remedy when symptoms do get better, since continuing with it there-after can cause them to recur.

Homeopathic remedies should not be touched with the hands or exposed to severe temperatures, which can "antidote" them or ren-der them ineffective. They can also be antidoted by coffee, alcohol, and camphor-containing products, including Vick's VapoRub, tiger balm, white flower oil, Noxzema creams, and BenGay. (If in doubt, read the label.) Homeopathic remedies should never be used along with steroid drugs, which work by an opposing system. Steroids sup-press the immune system's efforts to heal the body, while homeo-pathic remedies encourage it to regain its original vitality.

For more information about homeopathy, see sources in the Appen-dix. You may be able to find a practitioner in your area through the National Center for Homeopathy in Alexandria, Virginia. For more information about the medical self-care movement, see the maga-zine *Medical Self-Care*, now published in Healdsburg, California.

Homeopathic remedy with selected symptoms and indications

Aconite. Complaints begin after a fright or sudden shock; great thirst for cold drinks; anxiety states; panic attacks.

Apis. Marked aggravation from heat; flushes of heat; made better by cold applications; severe menstrual cramps.

Belladonna. Affected by change of temperature; all symptoms worse around menstrual period; intense heat in affected parts.

Calcarea carbonica. Heavy bleeding; uterine fibroids; sensation of inner trembling; perspiration on head or back of neck; craves sweets (pastries and ice cream).

Caulophyllum. Arthritis of fingers or toes, worse before menses; vaginitis; infertility; vaginal discharge; painful menstruation.

Chamomilla. Feet feel hot and must be put outside covers; oversensitive to pain; complaints of anger, great irritability, aversion to being touched.

Cimicifuga racemosa. Hot flashes worse at the onset of menstrual flow; severe headaches; changeable mood; talkative; jumps from one subject to the next.

Ignatia. Perspiration only on face; lump in throat; sighing; easily offended, defensive.

Kali carbonicum. Waking at night, especially 2 to 4 AM; wakes four hours after falling asleep.

Lachesis. Hot flashes better at onset of menstrual flow; suspicion, even paranoia; hot; aggravated by heat; irritable; jealous; depressed; flushes of heat.

Phosphorus. Tremendous thirst for cold drinks; bleeding bright red blood; uterine fibroids; uterine prolapse.

Pulsatilla. Weeps easily; headaches; worse with heat, exertion or after emotional stress; better in open air.

Sabina. Gushing flow of bright red blood, worse with motion; back pain with bleeding; thigh pain.

Sanguinara. Migraine headache on the right side; hot flashes; hay fever; heartburn.

Sepia. Involuntary weeping; symptoms worse from 2 to 4 PM or from 3 to 5 PM; flushes of heat with perspiration; worse at night.

Sulphur. Worse with heat; worse after bathing; craves sweets, chocolate, fats; insomnia.

(Continued on next page)

Figure 5: Popular Homeopathic Remedies for Hormonal Complaints

Homeopathic formulas for Menopause	Made by*
Menopause	Natra-Bio
Female Essentials	Longevity
Menocare	Boericke & Tafel
Hylaprin C #13	Hylands
Stramonium [for hot flashes only]	BHI
Rubus Idaeus	Dolisos
Homeopathic formulas for PMS	
Feminine	BHI
Menstrual	BHI
PMS	Boiron
Monthlies	Boericke & Tafel
Menstrual	Natra-Bio
Menstrusan	Bioforce
Menstrual Cramps	Dolisos
Fatigue	Dolisos

* See the Appendix.

Figure 5: Popular Homeopathic Remedies for Hormonal Complaints

Chapter Nine

Rebuilding Your Bones

Nature's above art....
—*King Lear*

Chinese and European herbal and homeopathic remedies have stood the test of time and are safe and effective for treating the symptoms of hormone imbalance. But do they protect women against cancer, heart disease, and osteoporosis? Studies that we'll look at in Chapter Fourteen show that these degenerative diseases are rare among older Chinese and Japanese women. (At least, they were when those women followed traditional diets and lifestyles.) But is it possible to prove a cause and effect relationship? And what if our energy systems have been out of balance for years? Will Chinese herbs and homeopathic remedies correct the problem at this late date? So far, these questions remain unanswered by Western science.

An herbal product that has been studied in the West for its effects on these degenerative conditions, however, is *natural* progesterone.

Plants produce molecules used for their own growth that are closely related to human hormones. Cholesterol derivatives called sapogenins that can easily be converted to progesterone for human use are made naturally by over 5000 plants.[1] The plant progesterone products on the market come from Mexican yams and soybeans. Only slight processing, not requiring the use of chemicals, is necessary to extract the sterols of these plants and make them exactly match the chemical composition of the body's own hormone. What is left after boiling is pure progesterone in powder form. This pure base is actually what drug companies use to produce patented synthetic progestins.

The problem with earlier attempts to use this natural progesterone in its pure form was that the liver converted it so rapidly for excretion that it couldn't be absorbed by the bloodstream or used by the body. To get it into the bloodstream efficiently, it had to be injected. The natural progesterone therapy first developed in the fifties by Katharina Dalton, M.D., involved injections, but it was expensive, cumbersome, and impractical. She later switched to a progesterone suppository, but it too had shortcomings. Less than one percent of the hormone is absorbed from some types of suppositories, and less than five percent absorption is usual.[2] More recently, an oral micronized pill was developed. ("Micronized" means the crystals have been smashed into a powder to aid absorption.) It was a definite advance, but like other oral hormones including Provera and Premarin, it must pass through the stomach and the liver, where much of the dose is lost. Adequate blood levels can be sustained only with large doses. The pills need to be taken several times a day, making them easy to forget. They also cause drowsiness in about 30 percent of women.[3] (This problem can be reduced by taking the full dose at night.)

These drawbacks were overcome in the seventies by the development of a technique by which the natural hormone could be suspended in vitamin E oil. This stable solvent allowed for efficient absorption of the hormone either through the stomach or the skin. Studies have shown that hormones are actually absorbed better through the skin than the stomach, substantially cutting dosage requirements.[4]

Natural progesterone in this transdermal form has been shown to reverse osteoporosis. In a study reported in the *International Clinical Review* in 1990 and in *Medical Hypotheses* in 1991, regular use of a natural progesterone cream not only retarded bone loss but actually restored the bones to their youthful thicknesses. The results were better than in studies with any other remedy, including estrogen.[5]

The study was begun in 1982 and was conducted by John R. Lee, M.D., an osteoporosis specialist with a clinical practice in Sebastopol,

California. The participants were 100 postmenopausal white women whose ages ranged from thirty-eight to eighty-three (average age sixty-five) and who were an average of sixteen years past menopause. They were followed for a minimum of three years, although most have been followed for much longer. After three years, bone density returned to safe levels in 100 percent of the patients treated; and in many of them, it stabilized at the levels of healthy thirty-five-year-olds.

The predicted change in bone density for the women over a three-year period was a loss of 4.5 percent. In fact, bone density *increased* by an average of 15.4 percent. Overall increases of 15 to 30 percent were common. Bones typically got 10 percent thicker in the first six to twelve months and increased 3 to 5 percent a year thereafter, and several patients' bone densities jumped 20 to 25 percent during the first year. This increase occurred regardless of age, in fact the patients who started out the worst improved the most.

Bone density also increased regardless of whether estrogen supplements accompanied the progesterone. A third of the women took no estrogen at all, and those who were already on it cut down to a fraction of what they'd been taking before. About 40 percent of these women later discontinued their estrogen use altogether.[6] That means about three-fourths of them did not need estrogen.

Dr. Lee now prescribes estrogen only for hot flashes and vaginal dryness, and then only after all else has failed. If natural progesterone alone doesn't eliminate or substantially reduce a patient's hot flashes, he first recommends other natural alternatives, including a diet rich in fresh vegetables and low in sugars and refined carbohydrates, aerobic exercise, and vitamin E. (See Chapters 14 and 15.)

The study suggested that natural progesterone is protective against not only osteoporosis but cancer and heart disease. Women who had fibroid tumors found the tumors did not enlarge, and after menopause they actually atrophied. Abnormal endometrial tissue reverted to normal. Women with fibrocystic breasts while on estrogen found relief when they switched to natural progesterone. Many of these women, said Dr. Lee, were spared having to have surgery for fibrocystic disease. Women whose blood pressures were high while on estrogen had normal blood pressures after switching to natural progesterone; and

HDL ("good") cholesterol levels did not fall, as they have with synthetic progestins.[7]

The beneficial effects of natural progesterone reported in this study have been confirmed in other research. Studies have shown that it significantly reduces hypertension in both men and women.[8] Like synthetic progestins, it maintains the uterine linings of women on estrogen in a condition that lowers endometrial cancer risk;[9] but unlike progestins, it has not been found to adversely affect cholesterol levels, and it has not produced the mood changes, weight gain, and other clinical side effects common on progestins.[10] Many of the women in Dr. Lee's osteoporosis study not only did not gain weight but actually lost it. They also reported they had more energy, and many volunteered the observation that their lost libido had returned.

The progesterone used was in the form of a cream applied to the skin. One-third to one-half of a one-ounce jar was used per month, applied to the softer skin under the arms or of the neck and face (since absorption is better through the softer skin), alternating sites each night. It was applied at bedtime for twelve days out of the month, or the last two weeks of estrogen use if estrogen was being used.

The women were also instructed to take the following measures known to counter osteoporosis. They were put on a low protein diet high in calcium-rich leafy green vegetables and low-fat cheeses. Red meat was limited to three times a week, and alcohol intake was limited. They were to avoid cigarettes, excess phosphates (especially in soft drinks), and certain drugs (e.g., excess thyroid hormone and corticosteroids). The following daily nutritional supplements were taken: 350 to 400 international units (IU) of vitamin D, 2000 milligrams (mg) of vitamin C in divided doses, 15 mg or 25,000 IU of betacarotene, and 800 to 1000 mg of calcium by diet and/or supplements. A modest exercise routine was also prescribed—20 minutes per day, or 30 minutes three times a week.

As a result of this program, osteoporotic pains were relieved, muscle and bone strength and mobility increased, osteoporotic fractures dropped to zero, and regular fractures healed unusually well. The study points to progesterone deficiency rather than estrogen deficiency as the major cause of menopausal osteoporosis. Estrogen's only known mechanism of action is to inhibit the osteoclasts, the cells that tear down old bone. That means all it can do is to slow bone loss. Progesterone stimulates the osteoblasts, the cells that make new bone.[11] The result is actual bone gain.

While some researchers have claimed that estrogen modestly increased bone mass in some studies, Dr. Lee points out that the estrogen in those studies was always accompanied by a progestin. Synthetic progestins have been shown to increase bone mass by as much as 5 to 6 percent.[12] This is a good result, but not so good as with natural progesterone; and progestins are accompanied by unwanted side effects not found with natural progesterone. In fact *no* unwanted side effects were reported by Dr. Lee's patients, not even monthly vaginal bleeding. Compare the side effects listed in the *Physician's Desk Reference* for Provera, summarized in Figure 6.[13]

Dr. Lee has recommended natural progesterone for thousands of women since 1982 and states that not only has he seen no significant side effects from its use, but bone loss has been reversed in every woman on whom he has tried it, so long as the other essential factors were included: proper diet and exercise, supplemental micronutrients, etc. While these other factors are necessary, they are not sufficient to explain the impressive results, which which were unique to his study and have not been equaled in studies not using natural progesterone.[14]

Dr. Lee's study was unique in another way: it was paid for by the women themselves. Most studies are funded by research grants from drug companies; but no drug company has been willing to finance osteoporosis studies involving natural progesterone, an unpatentable product. When Dr. Lee approached other researchers with what he considered to be overwhelming data on the benefits of the natural hormone, their response was, "That's interesting, but our research is limited to the scope of our grants." So his patients, who agreed that proving the benefits of natural progesterone to other women was a worthwhile objective, paid for their own bone density tests. Sixty-three of the women could afford these tests, at $150 each.

Dr. Lee tells of one seventy-two-year-old woman who had lost half her total bone mass and was severely osteoporotic when she started

Possible adverse reactions:
Breast tenderness and galactorrhea (milk secretion).
Sensitivity reactions (urticaria, pruritis, edema, rash).
Anaphylactoid reactions and anaphylaxis (severe acute allergic reactions).
Acne, baldness, hirsutism (abnormal hairiness).
Thrombophlebitis and pulmonary embolism.
Breakthrough bleeding, spotting, amenorrhea (missed periods), changes in menses.
Edema, weight change.
Cervical erosions and changes in cervical secretions.
Cholestatic jaundice.
Mental depression.
Fever.
Nausea.
Insomnia or somnolence.

When taken with estrogens, the following reactions have been observed:
Rise in blood pressure.
Premenstrual-like syndrome.
Headache, nervousness, dizziness, fatigue, changes in appetite, changes in libido.
Hirsutism and loss of scalp hair.
Skin irritations (erythema multiforme, erythema nodosum, hemorrhagic eruption, itching).

Precautions:
May cause fluid retention, epilepsy, migraine, asthma, cardiac or renal dysfunction; breakthrough bleeding or menstrual irregularities; depression.
The effect of prolonged use of this drug on pituitary, ovarian, adrenal hepatic, or uterine function is unknown.
May decrease glucose tolerance; diabetic patients must be carefully monitored.
May increase thrombotic disorders associated with estrogens.

Contraindications:
Thrombophlebitis, thromboembolic disorders, cerebral apoplexy, liver dysfunction or disease, known or suspected malignancy of breast or genital organs, undiagnosed vaginal bleeding, missed abortion, or known sensitivity.

Warnings:
May contribute to thrombophlebitis, pulmonary embolism, and cerebral thrombosis and embolism.
Increased risk of birth defects if taken during first four months of pregnancy.
Drug passes into breast milk; consequences unknown.
Beagle dogs given this drug developed malignant mammary nodules.
Discontinue if there is sudden or partial loss of vision.

Figure 6. Side Effects of Provera (Medroxyprogesterone Acetate)

on natural progesterone in 1982. Her bone density increased by 48 percent, to a level that was safe for her. She continued to get bone density tests every year, and every year her bone density remained at this high level. However, in 1993 her test came back 15 percent below what it had been the previous year. The spunky eighty-three-year-old woman was convinced the results were mistaken and had another test run. It confirmed that her bone density level was indeed still 48 percent higher than when she started using natural progesterone eleven years earlier.

Estrogen vs. progesterone

Dr. Lee's interest in natural progesterone was sparked by the research of biologist Raymond Peat, who studied the subject while doing his doctoral work on estrogen at the University of Oregon in the seventies. Dr. Peat found that estrogen given to laboratory animals significantly shortened their lives; but if the animals were given progesterone instead, they lived significantly longer than normal. Not only older animals but menopausal women seemed to show the effects of increased rather than decreased estrogen with age.[15] Estrogen and progesterone are antagonists with opposite effects. Dr. Peat's research revealed that aging effects come from estrogen, while anti-aging effects come from progesterone.

Although estrogen has been promoted as a "youth drug" that removes wrinkles, Dr. Peat cites research showing it actually advances aging in tissues, including the skin. It only appears to remove wrinkles, by causing the tissues to puff up with water. The prescription package insert states, "You may have heard that taking estrogens for years after menopause will keep your skin soft and supple and keep you feeling young." But it then concedes, "There is no evidence for these claims and such long-term estrogen use may have serious risks."

Natural progesterone balances out excess estrogen. It smoothes atrophied skin by increasing pigment cell size and branching, but it doesn't thicken youthful skin.[16]

Estrogen produces weight gain by causing cells to retain water and fat. In fact it's so effective for this purpose that it's given to chickens, turkeys, and cows just to fatten them up. It fills out the skin so the animal looks smooth and plump. Weight gain is also a common com-plaint of women on estrogen. Natural progesterone, on the other hand, causes weight loss, by improving the body's efficiency in burn-ing fuel for energy and by eliminating fluid. A natural diuretic, it competes with aldosterone for kidney receptors that cause water reten-tion, thus relieving edema (swelling).[17]

The greater cardiovascular health of premenopausal women with functioning ovaries has often been credited to estrogen, but Dr. Peat says that this effect is more likely to be a result of their high levels of progesterone. Excess estrogen results in excessive blood clotting, which *causes* heart attacks and strokes. Progesterone has been found to *prevent* stress-induced coronary blood vessel spasms, and it has been linked to delayed aging and longer lifespans.[18]

Even hot flashes, which most experts attribute to a shortage of estrogen, may in Dr. Peat's view be due to a shortage of progesterone relative to estrogen. He cites a study in which only ten percent of patients with menopausal symptoms including hot flashes could tell the difference between estrogen and a placebo. Other studies link menopausal flushing with an elevation of luteinizing hormone (LH). An elevation of LH, in turn, is linked with a lack of progesterone. Stress, which increases the incidence of hot flashes, causes a *rise* in estrogen. It also causes a loss of progesterone and thyroid hormone, which are "anti-estrogens."[19]

"These studies, and a few dozen others," says Dr. Peat, "have con-vinced me that the symptoms of menopause result mainly from a progesterone deficiency, relative to the estrogens. The 10 percent who really feel better from estrogen *possibly* have an estrogen defi-ciency, but this has not been determined, and several other things could account for the 'lift' they feel—for example, a *healthy* thyroid gland will respond to elevated estrogen with an increased output of thyroxin, which … might raise blood sugar, increase alertness, etc."[20]

What about the spark in your waning sex life that estrogen is said to supply? Again, progesterone is reported to work even better. Libido increases when you ovulate, because that's when your body wants to get the sperm and the egg together. The hormone the ovary makes when you ovulate is natural progesterone. On that theory, not only is progesterone a pro-libido hormone but estrogen is an *anti*-libido hormone.[21] Studies show estrogen doesn't actually restore libido. Apparently, it encourages sexual response simply by counteracting genital dryness, atrophy and hot flashes.[22] Masters, the sex researcher, reported that some women on estrogen-containing birth control pills lost their interest in sex and their ability to be aroused easily.[23]

"When one observes the many benefits from progesterone such as blood sugar normalization, more efficient utilization of fat for energy, bone formation, protection against cancer, enhancement of thyroid hormone, anti-depressant activity, and blockage of estrogen side effects," says Dr. Lee, "one must wonder why this valuable hormone has been so long neglected."[24]

Natural vs. synthetic progesterone

Why has it been? Probably because "progesterone" has been identified with the pharmaceutical versions. Synthetic progestins are chemically formulated from natural progesterone, but they are not its chemical equivalent. They can't be converted by the body into other steroid hormones as needed, and they're riddled with side effects.

Natural progesterone is converted by the adrenal glands into corticosteroids that aid in regulating blood sugar metabolism; but the adrenals can't use synthetic progestins for this essential conversion. The problem is compounded by the fact that when you take synthetics, your body produces less of the natural hormone; so the adrenals have nothing to convert into blood-sugar-regulating corticosteroids. The result can be a drop in blood sugar that brings on the fatigue and depression associated with hypoglycemia (low blood sugar). Symptoms may be made worse by salt buildup and fluid retention.[25]

As noted in Chapter Three, androgenic progestins can cause masculinization and the growth of unwanted facial hair, while estrogenic progestins can bring on fluid retention and edema (swelling). Natural progesterone does the reverse in each case. It reduces fluid retention by causing the body to hold potassium and throw off sodium, while synthetic progestins cause sodium to be retained. Sodium holds water in the tissues, causing puffiness and weight gain. Natural progesterone has also been used clinically to reverse the growth of facial hair. It does this in part by replacing the androgens older women synthesize to compensate for a progesterone deficiency.[26] The growth of facial hair and the loss of scalp hair can also result from impaired cortisone synthesis, and progesterone is a precursor of cortisone. By improving cortisone synthesis, supplementing with the natural hormone not only discourages unwanted facial hair but improves your ability to deal with stress—surgical, traumatic and emotional.[27]

If natural progesterone is so much better than synthetic versions, why isn't it in wider use? "The reluctance of contemporary medicine to adopt the use of natural progesterone is perplexing, to say the least," says Dr. Lee. "Since progesterone itself is readily derived from natural foods, one might wonder why the drug industry markets the synthetic compounds rather than natural progesterone, which has no known adverse side effects. It is difficult to ignore the conjecture that their synthetics are promoted simply because such compounds are patentable and thus potentially more profitable than natural progesterone."[28]

Another explanation may be that the benefits of the new natural progesterone products simply aren't well known. The FDA has required such caution in making claims that when we contacted three manufacturers of natural progesterone creams and oils for listing in the Appendix, two of them asked to be omitted.

Chapter Ten

Natural Progesterone Therapy from PMS to Menopause

Age cannot wither her, nor custom stale her infinite variety.
—*Anthony and Cleopatra*

The progesterone cream used by Dr. Lee is marketed by a company owned by nutritionist Bruce MacFarland. The process by which progesterone extracted from Mexican yams was suspended in vitamin E oil was developed in the seventies when Dr. Peat was working with Dr. MacFarland. (Dr. Peat now has his own company, called Kenogen.)

One of the first women to try the new product was MacFarland's daughter Sandy. She was only nineteen when her gynecologist recommended a hysterectomy. He said she had endometriosis and wouldn't be having children anyway. Endometriosis is a condition involving the abnormal growth of uterine tissue outside the uterus, causing chronic pelvic pain, disabling periods, internal scarring, and infertility. It affects five million American girls and women ranging in age from eleven to fifty and is a leading cause of hysterectomy. The Endometriosis Association considers the condition incurable.[1]

The MacFarlands declined the gynecologist's advice. Endometriosis can be stimulated by estrogen and is characterized by high blood levels of the hormone, indicating a hormone imbalance. Progesterone is a precursor to other hormones and normalizes their activity in the body. Sandy's father decided to try to correct her hormone imbalance with natural progesterone.

77

riment saved her uterus. Sandy had had only four peri-
vas sixteen, but she had a normal period the next month;
-nine she delivered a normal, healthy baby.

ne case points to a major advantage of natural progesterone over estrogen as hormone replacement therapy: it is safe for use before menopause, not only for the symptoms of perimenopause in the for-ties and fifties, but for PMS and other signs of hormone imbalance in younger women. Christiane Northrup, M.D., of the Women to Women Health Center in Yarmouth, Maine, recommends the cream for problems ranging from premenstrual migraine to hormone replace-ment for menopausal women. "I have been extremely impressed," she states, "and find it an extremely useful tool in my gynecological practice."

Hormone-related complaints that respond to natural progesterone before menopause include infertility, heavy menstrual bleeding, spot-ting between periods, amenorrhea (missed periods), and endometrial hyperplasia (an abnormal thickening of the uterine lining that can lead to uterine cancer). All of these conditions can be caused by low progesterone/estrogen ratios.[2]

Irregular or missed periods are often due to insufficient fat cells in which to store progesterone. The condition is sometimes seen in female professional athletes and in very thin women. It may result from very low cholesterol levels, since cholesterol is what hormones are made of. Natural progesterone has been reported to correct the condition by supplementing the body's insufficient progesterone storage.

Endometrial hyperplasia is an overgrowth of the uterine lining that can, if left untreated, develop into uterine cancer. It generally occurs among women who are not ovulating, either in their twen-ties and thirties or at menopause. Without ovulation, progesterone is not released. Excess endometrial tissue buildup is stimulated by excess estrogen, while insufficient progesterone prevents it from being uniformly shed. Estrogen replacement at menopause can exacerbate the condition.[3] The usual treatment is dilation and curettage (D&C), an operation involving scraping the uterine wall to rid it of excess endometrial buildup. The operation will relieve the problem temporarily, but the procedure has to be repeated. Natural progesterone has been reported to fix the problem permanently by addressing the cause rather than the effect.[4]

Natural progesterone and PMS

Natural progesterone's most popular use, however, is for treating PMS. It is best known and most widely used in the form of a micronized pill. Joel T. Hargrove, M.D., of Vanderbilt University, puts his success rate with PMS using micronized natural progesterone at 95 percent.[5] Niels Lauersen, M.D., professor of obstetrics and gynecology at New York Medical College, reports that 90 percent of his PMS patients who have tried natural progesterone have found relief.[6] Stephen Epstein, M.D., of the PMS Clinic in Seattle, reports an 85 to 90 percent success rate using the natural hormone. Dr. Peat, who uses the transdermal cream or oil, states that in the approximately 400 women he has observed, nearly all have found the appropriate amount to control their PMS symptoms.[7] Cheryl Harter, M.D., administrator of a PMS clinic in Phoenix, reports similar results.

Kathleen was one of these treatment successes. She suffered from devastating headaches every time she started her period. "I've had migraine-type headaches for all of my adult life," she reported. "I get sick to my stomach and sometimes vomit." She consulted chiropractors, a dentist for temporomandibular joint dysfunction (TMJ), an acupuncturist, a massage therapist, and an M.D., who recommended the Pill. "I've also taken a ton of aspirin over the last ten years. But once a headache starts, absolutely nothing helps. None of these treatments even made a dent in the frequency or intensity of the headaches." A month and a half after she began using a natural progesterone cream, her headaches disappeared.

Angie's problem was incapacitating fatigue. "I had a view of the outside world, clearly able to see other women who had the energy to do daily tasks and enjoy life. When faced with these same tasks my reactions were extreme fatigue," she recalls. "In recent years I have been unable to sleep through the night and unable to wake up in the morning." She tried every available form of therapy, conventional and alternative. Only natural progesterone cream reversed her symptoms. "Within four weeks," she said, "I began to sleep through the night, but the most noticeable improvement has been a new-found energy." Other symptoms that improved included stomach bloating, headaches, food cravings, and breast tenderness.

Despite these reports of good results, researchers are slow to credit progesterone therapy with helping PMS. The reason seems to be that the published studies involved other forms of the hormone besides either the natural micronized pills or the transdermal products. Controlled trials of several different synthetic progestins have failed to show any significant benefit on PMS symptoms.[8] Double-blind, crossover, placebo-controlled trials using vaginal or rectal suppositories have been equally unsuccessful at demonstrating benefit.[9] (Dr. Peat points out that the progesterone in suppositories using spermaceti wax goes out of solution very quickly, forming crystals that are essentially insoluble in body fluids.[10])

Only one controlled trial has reported significant improvements in PMS symptoms (anxiety, depression, swelling and hot flashes). It used natural progesterone in oral micronized form.[11] The transdermal cream doesn't seem to have been tested in reported studies; but practitioners stress that *only natural* progesterone works on PMS. Synthetic progesterone actually inhibits natural progesterone production and lowers its concentration in the blood.[12]

Natural progesterone and menopause

The side effects of synthetic progestins are are a major reason for the high dropout rate among women on HRT.

"Many women can take Premarin and still be healthy, just as some women can smoke and be healthy," comments Santa Monica acupuncturist Dr. Linda Forbes. "But I've never seen a healthy woman who was taking Provera. It's highly disruptive to the body's natural energy patterns and causes multiple distress syndromes."

Marie's was the extreme case. Her metabolism was so disturbed that her weight went up to 300 pounds. Donna was another synthetic progesterone casualty. She became too weak, tired, and depressed to function. These symptoms propelled her on an endless treadmill of doctor visits, pill popping, and hospitalizations that increased her dependence on drugs and destroyed her immune system.

Natural progesterone can solve this problem. In a study comparing effects and side effects in menopausal women given estrogen along with either natural oral progesterone or medroxyprogesterone acetate (Provera), those on natural progesterone reported *no* side effects. Their menopausal symptoms were better relieved and they had more favorable cholesterol levels than the women on Provera; and none wanted to discontinue hormone therapy, compared to forty percent on Provera.[13]

Studies of oral natural progesterone have confirmed that like synthetic progestins, it maintains the uterine linings of women on estrogen in a condition that lowers endometrial cancer risk. At the same time, it has not only eliminated the side effects of synthetics but lowered blood pressures and significantly reduced the rate of bleeding as compared to women on synthetic progestins.[14] Reviewers summarizing the literature in 1987 concluded that oral micronized progesterone "produces adequate plasma and tissue levels of progesterone," "reproduces the anti-estrogenic effect of the natural hormone on the endometrium," and "appears suitable for hormonal replacement therapy...."[15]

Whether natural progesterone is as effective as the pills hasn't been demonstrated in controlled trials, but if the hormone can be absorbed through the skin well enough to increase bone thicknesses by 15 to 30 percent—significantly more than with progestins—its absorption must be as effective as progestins in countering the tumor-stimulating effects of estrogen.

In Dr. Lee's experience, substituting natural for synthetic progesterone allows most women to reduce their estrogen dose by at least half; and after six months, women who are well past menopause can often give up estrogen altogether. For some women, natural progesterone controls hot flashes without the use of estrogen. Their bodies apparently synthesize estrogen from it as needed.

Take the case of Dorothy, whose menopausal symptoms dated back to 1975. "I had hourly violent hot flashes," she recalls. "They were overwhelming enough that I had to lie down for ten minutes." Dorothy's general health improved with vitamin therapy, but until she discovered natural progesterone cream, she still had hourly hot flashes. Now, she says, "I have the flashes only if I have over extended myself and then maybe two or three times a day—some days I don't have any." She adds, "What more can I say except 'get the word out'!"

Dr. Lee reports that few of the thousands of women he has treated with natural progesterone have suffered from hot flashes while they were using it. Of those who did, some resorted to estrogen; but others simply increased the dose of progesterone until relief was obtained. With synthetic patent remedies, dosage is limited because the drugs become more toxic the more you take; but he hasn't found natural progesterone to be toxic at any level.[16]

While that claim sounds overstated, hormone researcher Ray Peat confirms that it's supported by animal research. "Animals are generally more sensitive to progesterone than humans are," says Dr. Peat, "and in animals no toxic level has been found, except that in the highest doses it is anesthetic. In humans, even this effect has never been reported in the medical literature, and it is clearly anti-toxic in nature. Besides preventing acute poisoning of many kinds, it also reduces the incidence of birth defects and cancer."[17]

Relief of hot flashes from natural progesterone alone can take several months, since the hormone gets to the blood by way of the fat layer under the skin and builds up only gradually; but other natural remedies can be used to reduce hot flashes while the progesterone is kicking in. (See Chapters Seven, Eight, and Fifteen.) Trying this alternative before resorting to estrogen is worth the effort, not only because estrogen is a cancer promoter but because it's hard to get off it once you're on it. Withdrawing from natural progesterone is without reported side effects. After several months many women say their own hormones become normalized enough that they can cut down on the amount and eventually go without it.

Using natural progesterone for maximum benefit

Since manufacturers are restricted by the FDA from labeling their natural products with directions for use, you will need to consult a doctor (medical, Oriental medical, naturopathic, or homeopathic) to tailor your own individual program. Although your case should be evaluated individually, there are certain guidelines you and your

health care professional can follow for best results. Dr. Lee
following recommendations based on his clinical experie

He uses a natural progesterone cream called Pro-Gest made
by Transitions for Health (see the Appendix.) For reversing osteoporosis in postmenopausal women, he recommends using one-half
of a two-ounce jar per month for three weeks out of the month.
Abstaining for the fourth week allows the hormone receptor sites to
rebuild their sensitivity to the hormone. One ounce spread over three
weeks works out to about $\frac{1}{4}$ teaspoon per day. The first month or
two, while low progesterone levels are building up, this amount can
be doubled.

For women who want to substitute natural progesterone cream
for the progestin in their HRT, he suggests continuing to use half the
usual dose of the synthetic along with the cream for the first two
months. Again, this is because the natural hormone when absorbed
through the skin gets to the blood by way of body fat, and two or
three months may be required to attain proper blood levels.

For prompt response in acute cases (hot flashes or migraine
headaches), natural progesterone is available in an under-the-tongue
liquid or oil form. It is quickly absorbed through the mucus mem-
branes of the mouth, avoiding digestion.[18] In fact Dr. Peat recommends using this oil, which is more concentrated than the cream, on
the skin. "Natural progesterone is not known to have any side effects,
except for alteration of the menstrual cycle and production of eupho-
ria until doses of several grams per day are reached, at which point
its anesthetic property begins to appear," Dr. Peat reports. "The basic
procedure should be to use it in sufficient quantity to make the symptoms disappear, and to time its use so that menstrual cycles are not
disrupted."[19]

More natural progesterone is required for PMS than for osteoporosis, because the hormone has to counter an excess of estrogen in
women who are still menstruating. To treat PMS, a full two-ounce
jar of the cream is recommended per month to start with. Progesterone should be begun on day 10 or 12 of the cycle (counting the
first day of menstruation as day 1), finishing on day 25 or 26. That's
a bit more than $\frac{1}{2}$ teaspoon per day. Requirements, however, are very

individual. Dr. Lee recommends experimenting to find the right amount. For one of the authors (Ellen), a mere $\frac{1}{8}$ to $\frac{1}{16}$ teaspoon daily for half the month seems to be enough to produce a pleasant stimulating effect on energy level and sex drive without side effects.

While no serious or irreversible side effects are reported in the medical literature from natural progesterone, some women do report minor reactions as their bodies adjust to the new regime, including drowsiness, breast tenderness, water retention, and spotting. Dr. Lee advises his patients to wait three months before they tell him how they feel. After that period, he says, he's had no complaints.

Drowsiness, he suggests, results in women who actually need sleep. Many of us frantically push ourselves through overcrowded schedules, becoming tight and tense, rendering the sleep we do get less than refreshing. Natural progesterone lets us finally relax. For once, the body prevails over the frenetic schedule, coaxing us into bed. After a few good nights' sleep, women report they are energized rather than made drowsy by the natural hormone.

Breast tenderness, suggests Dr. Lee, is caused not by the progesterone itself but by an initial estrogen effect, as the estrogen receptors are enhanced and more estrogen is allowed into the cells. This effect goes away as progesterone levels continue to rise.

Altering the timing of your monthly periods can result if you don't keep to your natural cycle. You should take the hormone from the approximate time of ovulation until two or three days before your menstrual period is expected. On the twenty-fifth day, progesterone levels fall off naturally, signalling the pituitary to tell the uterus to flush its built-up lining in menstruation.

Even if you do keep to this timing, your periods may be altered with first progesterone use. After the second or third month, however, regularity should return. In fact, says Lila Nachtigall, M.D., "If you take progesterone, you will have regular periods until you run out of estrogen." This reassuring regularity can also eliminate the nagging question that accompanies missed periods, "Is is menopause or am I pregnant?"[20]

Transdermal natural progesterone has the advantage over the pill that much lower amounts are required to get an effect, but pharmacist and homeopath Lynne Walker has seen cases of allergic skin reactions to the cream. However, she notes that any remedy applied to the skin will have this effect in a small number of users. Reactions to natural progesterone cream are substantially less likely than to the estrogen patch, which continuously irritates the skin and deprives it of oxygen.[21]

All of these reactions to natural progesterone are minor compared to those reported for synthetic progestins. Compare the side effects and cautions listed in the *PDR* for Provera (medroxyprogesterone acetate), summarized in Figure 6 in the last chapter. How much Provera differs from the natural hormone is shown by the fact that if given to a pregnant woman, the drug can kill the fetus or cause its deformity. The body's own progesterone, by contrast, is the hormone of gestation: it promotes the growth of the developing fetus. In a study conducted by Katharina Dalton, M.D., natural progesterone was given to women to prevent toxemia of pregnancy and their offspring were followed to adulthood. The children actually scored better on tests and achieved higher levels of education than matched controls.[22]

Besides Pro-Gest, natural plant progesterone creams on the market include a similar product made by Dr. Peat's company Kenogen, and Progonol made by Bezwecken. Natural progesterone in pill form is available from Madison Pharmacy Associates and Women's International Pharmacy. (See the Appendix.)

Chapter Eleven

If You Need Estrogen

I know I have the body of a weak and feeble woman, but I have
the heart and stomach of a king, and of a king of England too.
—Queen Elizabeth I (1533–1603)

Having exhausted the warnings and precautions against taking estrogen, let's look at the woman with a true estrogen shortage. Indications include hot flashes or vaginal dryness that don't respond to other
remedies. In Dr. Lee's study of osteoporotic postmenopausal women,
about 25 percent needed estrogen by those standards, while Dr. Peat
cites research putting the figure at 10 percent.[1]

After your hysterectomy

Women whose hormone output has been curtailed abruptly and prematurely by hysterectomy/oophorectomy are prime candidates for
ERT. "Hot flashes and heavy sweating in hysterectomized-oophorec-
tomized women are more severe and more sudden in onset than those
seen in natural menopause," says Vicki Hufnagel, M.D., author of *No
More Hysterectomies*. "For some women, hot flashes and night sweats
increase significantly after hysterectomy, even when the ovaries are
preserved."[2]

These hot flashes need immediate treatment, but prescription
estrogen isn't the only choice. Dr. Walker has helped hundreds of
menopausal women overcome their symptoms, and unless they were
already on estrogen, she has so far succeeded in relieving their hot

flashes with Oriental herbs and other plant-based natural products. Traditional Chinese herbal formulas come in balanced combinations that avoid the side effects and risks of ERT.

Sarah came to Dr. Walker five months after she'd had a hysterectomy/oophorectomy at the age of thirty-six. Because she'd had a Pap smear indicating cervical cancer, her doctor refused to give her estrogen. He said she would just have to suffer with her hot flashes, and this she was indeed doing. She was nervous, anxious, tired, unable to sleep, and had gained substantial weight, largely from water retention. Dr. Walker gave her the Chinese herbal formula *Quiet Contemplative*. (See Figure 3 in Chapter 7.) Sarah was amazed at the results. Not only did her hot flashes disappear but many of her other bothersome symptoms did too.

Natural progesterone is another possibility. Estrogen from external sources is necessary only if the body is unable to make a sufficient supply from this precursor hormone. Natural progesterone has been reported to work without estrogen even on the menopausal symptoms following surgical menopause in some cases. However, relief usually takes longer than in cases of natural menopause (maybe one to six months).[3]

Even if you are already taking estrogen after a hysterectomy, you don't need to stay on it forever. Health writer John McDougall, M.D., states that after about age forty-five, when estrogen production would have fallen off anyway, you can gradually wean yourself from it.[4] Again, the problem is that it's hard to get off estrogen once you start. Supplementing with estrogen raises the "set-point" below which you'll experience hot flashes. When you're withdrawing from estrogen, hot flashes can be worse than before you started taking it. It's important to wean yourself from estrogen gradually. Taking natural progesterone along with it can help you decrease the dose without uncomfortable symptoms. (See Chapter Ten.)

Women who have had a hysterectomy typically aren't given progestins along with estrogen because they don't have to worry about uterine cancer. However, *natural* progesterone can still be useful to these women, not only to help them decrease the need for estrogen but to preserve their bones. Women taking estrogen merely lose bone less rapidly than other women; but natural progesterone actually increases bone density.[5] Unlike synthetic progestins, it may also reduce breast cancer risk. Progesterone combined with estrogen blocks estrogen receptors in the breasts and ovary and seems to prevent the development of cancer sites outside the uterus.[6] Several practitioners have reported that when natural progesterone cream has been applied directly to breast tumors, they have shrunk.[7]

Estrogen from plants

For women who need estrogen and progesterone but have trouble with the prescription versions, both hormones in their HRT can be replaced with natural plant products. Both plants and animals produce hormones that regulate cell metabolism and growth; and estrogen, like progesterone, can be found in both. The sterols of plants like soybeans and yams are the basis from which many cheap, commercially-available hormones are made. Studies establishng the advantages of natural plant estrogens are underway. Preliminary results of some of these studies are discussed in the Introduction.[8]

Substituting plant for prescription hormones worked for Helen. Without natural progesterone and estrogen creams, she said, she was unable to function. "There are no side effects—no hot flashes, no fluctuating mood swings. I am especially thankful for the fact that they are both natural products—as I am unable to use any other."

Jesse Hanley, M.D., who practices in Malibu, California, has had good success treating her patients for hot flashes using a natural estrogen/progesterone cream called OstaDerm, made by Bezwecken. Both hormones come from Mexican yams.

The cream contains all three endogenous forms in which estrogen is found naturally in the body, estrone (E1), estradiol (E2), and estriol (E3). They're in a ratio of 1:1:8, with the 80 percent portion being estriol. Estriol is not used in estrogen replacement pills in the United States, but research studies suggest it may be a safer form of estrogen than the estrone that predominates in Premarin or the estradiol found in the patch (Estraderm).[9]

Estriol is the least active form of estrogen and is considered in this country to be weak and ineffective; but studies from Europe, where it is widely used, suggest it's just as effective as E1 and E2 if given in adequate doses. Its major advantage is that while E1 and E2 have been implicated as cancer promoters, E3 may actually be protective against the disease.

The healthy liver breaks down the carcinogenic forms E1 and E2 into the less active E3 form; but if the liver is weak and inactive, E1 and E2 will lodge in the estrogen receptors of the breast and uterus, increasing the risk of estrogen dependent cancers, fibrocystic breast disease, and ovarian cysts. E3, which retains its unique identity in the body even when taken orally, is thought to prevent this result by lodging in these estrogen receptors and keeping the dangerous forms out. At least, that was the conclusion of researchers writing in the *Journal of the American Medical Association* in 1978.[10] While that was more than a decade ago, more recent research is lacking. Much of the original estrogen research was sponsored by Wyeth-Ayerst, which has no further incentive to look at alternatives since its Premarin now has a monopoly on the oral conjugated estrogen market.

Though estriol is thought to actually protect against cancer, this effect has not yet been proved to the FDA; so the manufacturer still advises against its use by women with estrogen contraindications. Dr. Hanley cautions that in her experience, the progesterone in the 1-1-8 plant hormone formulation is insufficient to balance out its estrogen content for many women; so she recommends natural progesterone cream along with it. She also stresses that plant estrogens, like animal estrogens, should be used only under the guidance of a competent health care professional. Any estrogen if used improperly can cause painful, tender breasts and unwanted bleeding. Regular examinations and annual Pap smears are still required.

Other estrogen options

Transitions for Health also makes a plant extract that contains natural estrogen. Called Es-Gen, it mimics Premarin in consisting primarily of estrone (E1), but the plant version is extracted from soybeans as sitosterol. Allergic reactions have been reported from Premarin, which contains an estrogen found naturally only in horses, as well as additives necessary to make it a tablet. But so far, no allergic reactions have been reported from natural plant estrone cream, which can be used as a more natural substitute. It too, however, should be avoided by women with estrogen contraindications.

On the other hand, while we're waiting for definitive research on plant estrogens, some holistic practitioners feel that Premarin remains the safer choice, since it comes in an oral form that allows for more accurate measurement than transdermal forms. Other oral prescription estrogens include Estrace, which consists of micronized estradiol; and Ogen, which consists of purified crystalline estrone.

Another alternative is the transdermal estrogen patch (Estraderm), but many holistic practitioners warn against it. It contains estradiol (E2), the form of estrogen found by Swedish researchers to be the most likely to produce breast cancer;[11] and absorption rates are hard to control, making overdose a serious risk. Skin irritation is experienced by about eleven percent of women on the patch, and it's more expensive than the pill. Some women also complain of an uncomfortable feeling of fullness and other side effects not common with estrone. The patch currently comes in only two strengths, reducing the likelihood of finding the appropriate dose for your particular needs.[12]

An alternative for women who can't or don't want to take conventional doses of estrogen may be to take it in homeopathic doses. (See Chapter Eight.) Like all homeopathic versions of prescription drugs, the FDA has made homeopathic estrogen a prescription-only item. However, it is without long-term risks, since like other homeopathic remedies, it's so diluted as to contain virtually none of the estrogen it's made from. Little information is available on homeopathic estrogen because it has too little profit potential to be worth investigating and promoting; but practitioners who use it report that it's generally effective for women who need it.[13]

Estrogen for atrophic vaginitis: Dryness, itching, burning

"I survived hot flashes without estrogen," Katherine confided, "but I need something for my vagina. It's dry and itchy and painful; and it's shrunk up so much I can't have intercourse. My husband's afraid to even try, for fear he'll hurt me. But our relationship isn't the same without sex."

Lack of vaginal lubrication during intercourse means hormone levels are dropping. It can be one of the first symptoms of menopause. Classic symptoms of vaginal atrophy are dryness, irritation, burning, and a feeling of pressure. There may also be a yellowish discharge. The vagina gets progressively shorter and narrower, its skin tissue thins, and its muscular layer is replaced with fibrous tissue. The vagina shrivels and shrinks and loses its flexibility, while the labia become small, colorless, and flat.[14]

The vagina also becomes susceptible to infection. This is because its thin walls lack the normal secretions that cleanse the vaginal tissues. Vaginal pH rises (meaning it becomes more alkaline instead of the normal acid), allowing undesirable bacteria to replace the friendly bacterial flora. The result can be urinary tract infections. Antibiotics are usually prescribed; but since the problem is the alkalinity of the vagina, the infections tend to recur, leading to long-term drug use that can be dangerous and expensive.[15] Many physicians resort to chronic suppressive therapy with sulfonamides (sulfa drugs), which can produce life threatening complications.[16]

An alternative approach is hormone treatment. In a 1988 University of Florida Medical School study, when postmenopausal women with a history of recurrent infection and antibiotics were treated with estrogen, vaginitis was cured and urinary tract infections went away for good. The estrogen worked by restoring the normal vaginal flora and pH.[17]

An interesting side issue was the form in which the hormone should be given. At first, the women took it by mouth; but they were already past menopause and were upset by the return of their periods, painful enlargement of the breasts, and nausea. Some of the women were therefore switched to a vaginal estrogen cream taken twice weekly. The cream, which avoided passage through the digestive tract, proved to be just as effective as the pills without their unpleasant side effects.

Hormone therapy can help in cases not only of vaginal infection but of vaginal dryness and atrophy. Women's complaints in general, and this one in particular, are only now beginning to be researched, so studies are few and far between; but research is available from Europe. In a European study reported in 1991, twenty postmenopausal women (average age seventy-three) were treated with oral estrogen in the form of estriol. When their flora and epithelial cells were compared to those of twenty untreated women of similar age and twenty healthy younger women (average age twenty-eight), they more nearly resembled those of the younger women than of the untreated postmenopausal women.[18]

A 1991 Norwegian review concluded that estriol is a safe, cheap and effective therapy for the symptoms of estrogen deficiency after menopause, including atrophy of the vagina, urethra and bladder, urinary tract infections, and abnormal function of the lower urinary tract. The researchers found that estriol had no metabolic effects or serious side effects at recommended doses and was safe for use long-term.[19]

Oral estriol is not available in this country, but estriol is the major estrogen component in OstaDerm estrogen/progesterone cream. While the OstaDerm transdermal cream is not designed for vaginal use, Bezwecken makes a 1-1-8 estrogen/progesterone suppository that is. David Shefrin, N.D., a naturopathic doctor in Beaverton, Oregon, who specializes in menopausal and premenstrual complaints, uses this cream for severe atrophic vaginitis. He observes, "It has always amazed me how easily the vaginal problems can be reversed. Women whose vaginas bled just with the introduction of a small speculum or from taking a Pap smear return literally after six weeks with a moist, pink, youthful vagina. Not all cases can be completely reversed in just six weeks, however. In those women with profound atrophy, the process may take a few months. Prognosis then depends on how great the loss of estrogen was and for how long. So it's very important to educate these women early on."[20]

Studies show that vaginal estrogen creams are as effective as oral estrogen. In fact absorption of estrogen through the vagina is so efficient that researchers have been concerned that women would run the same cancer risks with vaginal creams as with oral estrogen.[21] Preliminary research discussed in the Introduction indicates that plant estrogens not only aren't cancer-promoting but may be cancer-protective. However, it is still important to take natural progesterone along with vaginal estrogen cream, since the progesterone affords protection against bone loss. Moreover, the favorable research results are merely preliminary. The guidance of a competent licensed practitioner should still be sought when using estrogen, whatever its source. John Lee, M.D., recommends natural progesterone cream alone applied vaginally for vaginal complaints.

The natural way to maintain vaginal lubrication is to remain sexually active; but as women like Katherine would protest, lack of vaginal lubrication can keep you from being sexually active. Besides the hormone creams, non-hormone vaginal lubricants and moisturizers are available. A vaginal suppository called Replens is effective but expensive. Cheaper options are K-Y jelly and Mennen's Baby Magic. However, all of these products contain mineral oil, which blocks pores and congests tissue, is difficult for the body to dispose of, and tends to be allergenic. A product that is petroleum-free is Women's Health Institute Lubricating Gel (see the Appendix).

Another natural product that studies show to be effective in relieving atrophic vaginitis is vitamin E. You can insert the capsules vaginally, take them by mouth, or open them up and apply the oil directly to the vaginal tissues.

Chapter Twelve

Preserving Your Female Organs: Alternatives to Surgery

It should be forbidden and severely punished to remove cancer by cutting, burning, cautery and other fiendish tortures. It
is from nature that the disease arises and from nature comes
the cure, not from the physicians.
                                        —Paracelsus (1493–1541)

We've seen that one risk you run when you take estrogen is the development of fibroid tumors precipitating hysterectomy. Fibroids are non-
malignant masses of connective tissue that tend to grow on the wall
of the uterus before menopause, when estrogen secretion dominates.
After menopause, when estrogen secretion falls off, these tissue lumps
normally atrophy away; but this can't happen if estrogen is supplemented artificially. Estrogen is a tumor stimulant. It encourages both
uterine fibroid tissue and breast tissue growth. If estrogen is supplied
after menopause, fibroid tumors will be stimulated to grow. Although
these fibroids usually remain non-malignant, they can cause excessive
menstrual bleeding and pelvic pain, resulting in hysterectomy.[1]

Fibroid tumors are, in fact, the most common reason given for
this surgery. More than 40 percent of women over fifty have these
benign growths; and from 1982 to 1984, more than half a million
uteri were removed to excise them. "Many of these surgeries are carried out on women in their twenties and thirties who have no children," observes Los Angeles gynecologist Vicki Hufnagel, M.D. "They
are not told that they have options."[2]

95

Tumor-shrinking herbs

Co-author Lynne Walker was one of these statistics. As noted in the Introduction, she was only thirty-three when she was told she needed a hysterectomy because a large fibroid tumor was growing in her uterus. Conventional wisdom says that fibroids cannot be dissolved. They can only be removed.[3] Before Dr. Walker agreed to surgery, however, she was determined to explore the alternatives. She went to an acupuncturist who gave her Chinese herbs, acupuncture, and homeopathic remedies. When these resolved Dr. Walker's problem without surgery, she was so impressed that she broadened her field of expertise from pharmacy to Chinese medicine and homeopathy. Since then, she has seen Oriental and Western herbal remedies help shrink the tumors of her patients.

A European herbal formula that was particularly promising was Petasan, an over-the-counter product made by Dr. A. Vogel's Swiss herbal company Bioforce. Petasan is composed of a combination of the herbs mistletoe and butter bur. In 1991, at the recommendation of European homeopath Jan DeVries, Dr. Walker gave it to six women with fibroid tumors. Within a week, all six reported that their bleeding and other painful symptoms had subsided. Two of the women's fibroids had shrunk from grapefruit size to the size of a walnut, and all of the women were doing well, when the FDA banned the product's further sale, saying that Petasan was not one of its accepted herb products. Although the formula is not now available in the United States or Canada, its individual ingredients (mistletoe and butter bur) can be purchased in Canada and other countries.

Dr. Walker has also seen homeopathic remedies shrink tumors. Trudy's was one such case. Trudy came to Dr. Walker with a hard lump in the middle of her tongue. Her own doctor told her she needed surgery and had scheduled an operation for a month later. In the meantime, Dr. Walker gave her a homeopathic remedy called Calcarea Fluorica 12x. When Trudy's surgeon looked into her mouth during her pre-operative exam, the lump had disappeared. Trudy then announced that she had been using homeopathic remedies. Although the doctor's reaction was simply annoyance at the disruption in his surgery schedule, Trudy herself was delighted. (Calcarea Fluorica is also very effective on ganglion cysts and bone spurs.)

Oriental herbs can also be effective against tumors. In a recent study, proteins extracted from Chinese medicinal herbs were shown to selectively injure tumor cell lines while preserving normal cell lines. That made the herbs superior to conventional cytotoxic ("cell-killing") chemotherapy, which kills normal along with aberrant cells.[4]

Chinese herbal products useful for shrinking unwanted growths include *Laminaria 4* (for fatty type swellings), *Zedoaria Tablets* (for hard masses), and *Chih-ko and Curcuma* (for phlegm or blood stagnation, considered in Chinese medicine to be the cause of many fibroids). They are all made by Seven Forests (see Appendix A).

Alhough the natural remedies discussed here are safe, you should not attempt self-treatment. Fewer than .2 percent of fibroid tumors are found to be malignant, but that remains a possibility.[5] If you have symptoms suggesting fibroids—including abdominal swelling, pelvic or back pain, heavy or irregular bleeding, painful periods, constipation, pressure on the bladder, or frequent urination—see a gynecologist. If you are interested in exploring natural remedies, see an Oriental medical, homeopathic, or naturopathic physician.

Natural progesterone and tumors

Hormone researcher John Lee, M.D., maintains that uterine fibroids, breast fibrocysts, and painful breast swelling can be both prevented and treated with natural progesterone. Both conditions are common in the estrogen-dominant phase of perimenopause. Supplementing with natural progesterone before menopause can prevent them from developing; while supplementing with it after menopause is an effective way to protect yourself against bone loss while avoiding the risk of fibroid development that accompanies estrogen.[6]

Dr. Lee cites the case of a former patient who telephoned to say she had developed a large fibroid tumor. Her gynecologist, concerned that its rapid growth suggested cancer, recommended immediate removal of her uterus and ovaries. Should she agree?

Dr. Lee recommended natural progesterone cream, and the patient took his advice. When she returned to her gynecologist a month later, the tumor was about 10 percent smaller. The gynecologist continued to recommend surgery, while Dr. Lee continued to recommend natural progesterone. The patient continued to follow Dr. Lee's recommendations.

After three months, the tumor was 25 percent reduced. Six months later (ten months from when she began using natural progesterone), it was gone. This simple treatment allowed the woman to avoid hysterectomy and preserve her uterus and ovaries.

Dr. Lee has also successfully treated ovarian cysts with natural progesterone. Most of these cysts, he says, are due to failed ovulation. When natural progesterone is supplied, each ovary thinks the other is supplying it, and they take a rest.

He tells of a patient who was troubled with both ovarian cysts and a fibroid tumor. After three months' treatment with natural progesterone, the cysts disappeared and the fibroid was substantially smaller. Despite these dramatic effects, the patient's gynecologist refused to believe that natural progesterone had done it, since he was not convinced that progesterone could be effectively absorbed from a cream through the skin. Dr. Lee therefore recommended a test to determine the patient's blood progesterone levels. Normal levels for a menstruating woman are in the ten to twenty range; but this woman was well past menopause and her ovaries had quit producing hormones, so her progesterone level should have been near zero. In fact, it was forty—twice that of a healthy young woman.

Breast fibrocysts also respond to natural progesterone. The condition is characterized by an overgrowth of fibrous tissue and a higher level of circulating estrogen, indicating a hormonal imbalance. In Dr. Lee's clinical experience, these breast lumps usually disappear after two or three months of natural progesterone treatment. "Very few things in medicine are this easy to treat," he observes. "It is staggering to consider the many women who suffer needlessly from these problems."[7]

Surgical reconstruction

Even if surgery is required for fibroids or uterine prolapse, there may be alternatives to removing the female organs. Vicki Hufnagel, M.D.,

98

author of *No More Hysterectomies*, favors a surgical re-sectioning of the uterus called "female reconstructive surgery."

The procedure involves opening the abdomen with a bikini-type incision and lifting the uterus out for complete inspection. The tissue connected to the uterus is clamped off with a special clamp, and the drug Pitressin is injected to stop the flow of blood. The idea is to allow maximum surgical time without bleeding. Tumors are then removed or, in the case of uterine prolapse, the ligaments and organs are restructured and resuspended. Dr. Hufnagel learned this procedure from Peter Taleghany, M.D., with whom she worked for many years. Dr. Taleghany has successfully performed thousands of these surgeries since 1955 and is currently practicing in the Westwood area of Los Angeles.

Dr. Hufnagel maintains that up to 90 percent of the hysterectomies currently performed might be avoided if other options were explored. Even fibroid tumors that are growing rapidly are not, in her view, usually grounds for removing the uterus. Non-malignant fibroids can be surgically removed without removing the organ.

Dr. Hufnagel helped conduct a statistical survey of American hysterectomies performed between 1965 and 1984 published by the U.S. Department of Health and Human Services. It found that only 10.5 percent of these operations were medically indicated and necessary due to cancer. The others were elective surgeries performed for a variety of reasons, including sterilization and uterine prolapse. The reason for the surge in hysterectomies is a matter of speculation, but the explanation she suggests is economic: the operation is the bread-and-butter surgery of OB/GYNs, who are backing away from obstetrics because of increasing medical malpractice liability. They're leaning toward the safer, easier hysterectomy, the most frequently performed major gynecological surgery.[8]

The thyroid connection

The heavy and irregular menstrual bleeding that can signal a uterine tumor can also be a symptom of something else: hormone imbalance from an underactive thyroid gland. In the opinion of hormone researcher Ray Peat, "a physician who advocates removal of the uterus for excessive bleeding, without first trying thyroid therapy, is not practicing medicine properly."[9] An impaired thyroid can also impair the effectiveness of natural progesterone. Before you resort either to estrogen or to hysterectomy, it's a good idea to have your thyroid function tested.

Hypothyroidism (a deficiency of thyroid hormone) can cause not only menstrual problems but weight gain, sluggishness, cold extremities, anemia, headaches, and an increased susceptibility to infection, heart disease, cancer, and premature aging. It causes stomach acid and other digestive juices to be in short supply and intestinal movements to be weak, so gas and constipation are common. A woman with this condition can be malnourished even on a good diet, because she isn't properly assimilating her food. She can also gain substantial weight even when she is honestly (as she claims) eating almost nothing, because she isn't burning her calories efficiently.

A simple way to find out whether your thyroid levels are low is to check your body temperature when you wake up in the morning. A temperature below 98 degrees and a slow pulse may be indicative of hypothyroidism.

Another home test, recommended by Dr. MacFarland and available from Transitions for Health, involves the application of tincture of iodine to the skin. The tincture works both as a test of thyroid function and as a treatment.

"T-3" and "T-4" tests are thyroid tests often used by doctors, but they aren't very reliable. The Thyroid Stimulating Hormone (TSH) test is a more useful indicator of thyroid function. A high TSH test means the pituitary is signalling the thyroid to make more thyroid hormone. A low TSH test means you have enough or even too much thyroid hormone.[10]

If you need thyroid therapy, it should be prescribed by a medical professional. *Excess* thyroid supplementation can be harmful. Excess thyroid hormone stimulates the osteoclasts, the cells that tear down or resorb bone. Bone resorption should be in balance with bone formation. An excess of resorption over formation results in bone loss.[11]

The usual thyroid medication is synthetic thyroxine (levothyroxine or Synthroid), but it has drawbacks. The same stress that blocks the thyroid can block conversion of the synthetic hormone to T3 (triiodothyronine), the form in which thyroid hormone is most active in the body.[12] A better, more natural option is Armour Thyroid, which is standardized to government specifications. It used to be available in health food stores but has now been made a prescription item. In the case of thyroid products, it's best to avoid generic "equivalents," which aren't really equivalent to the government-standardized originals.

Before supplementing with thyroid hormone, non-drug means of stimulating the thyroid should be tried, including acupuncture, homeopathy, and nutritional supplements. Thyroid function is dependent on a balance of two trace minerals, manganese and iodine. Hypothyroidism could be due to a shortage of either. Herbs useful as thyroid stimulants include dulse and kelp. For homeopathic and other natural remedies, consult a homeopathic, naturopathic, or Chinese medical physician.

Chapter Thirteen

Natural Mood Elevators

Women's moods found treatable; still no hope for men.
—Michelle Harrison, M.D.[1]

Thyroid and other natural hormones can relieve not only the physical but the emotional symptoms of hormone imbalance—anxiety and depression. "When I have watched suicidal women using thyroid and progesterone," says Dr. Peat, "there is a transformation (under an hour with progesterone, a few hours or longer with thyroid) from weeping to smiling and laughing; they speak of unbearable pain being replaced by pleasure.[2]"

Estrogen can have similar benefits for menopausal women. Author Lonnie Barbach quotes Dr. John Arpels: "I can't tell you how many women I've gotten off of Prozac, which their internists prescribed for midlife crisis, when what they were experiencing was really an estrogen phenomenon. Most physicians just don't understand this at all."[3]

Depression is a common complaint of women undergoing the Change. Often the mood is inexplicable. Virginia remembers the time her husband came home to find her collapsed in tears. "What's wrong?", he asked in alarm. "Nothing's wrong," sobbed his normally even-tempered wife. "I'm just upset at being upset!"

Psychological factors—loss of the ability to bear children, the empty-nest syndrome, and uncertainty about what to do for the next thirty years—used to be blamed for menopausal depression. These may indeed be factors, but the condition has now also been linked to hormone imbalances. To the extent that depression has physical roots, it can be corrected by physical means. Helpful therapies include not only hormones but herbs that restore hormone balance, nutritional supplements, and dietary change.

Hormones as uppers

Low progesterone levels can cause depression by causing low blood sugar and water retention. Supplementing with the natural hormone can correct these imbalances in premenopausal as well as postmenopausal women. "Cyclic edema, depression, and migraine are, in my experience, always stopped by progesterone," says Dr. Peat. "Sexual functions are often improved."[4]

Victoria suffered from severe depression. She also had migraine headaches, aches in her pelvis that were so acute she thought she had arthritis, severe fatigue, severe memory loss, and continual bouts with colds and flu-like symptoms. These problems were all reversed by natural progesterone, which she called "a godsend."

For menopausal women, natural progesterone can also alleviate the hot flashes that keep them up half the night. Sleep deprivation can be devastating to the psyche, causing chronic fatigue, depression, and an inability to function.

Estrogen, too, can relieve menopausal depression, anxiety, and headaches. Partly this is due to its beneficial effect on the hot flashes that are devastating to sleep, but research also links it to the increased availability of L-tryptophan triggered by the hormone. L-tryptophan is an amino acid that breaks down in the brain into other substances, including the mood-elevating neurotransmitter serotonin, a natural "upper" that mediates depression. L-tryptophan levels have been found to be low in depressed menopausal women. These levels are brought back to normal by estrogen treatment.[5]

The tryptophan and Prozac controversies

In theory, you could avoid the side effects of estrogen by supplementing with L-tryptophan itself. L-tryptophan is the most effective serotonin producer currently known, and for nearly half a century it was used as a safe and natural alternative to pharmaceutical tranquilizers. It was inexpensive and, until recently, was readily available. But in 1989, after decades of incident-free use, the FDA removed the product from the market.

The ban was precipitated by reports of serious side effects and deaths, tragedies traced to contamination in the manufacturing process used by a particular Japanese manufacturer from late 1988 to early 1989. Oddly, the manufacturer had changed three separate production factors at the same time, a move at variance with the usual strict quality control maintained by the Japanese. The process producing the contaminated by-products involved genetic engineering. A study reported in the *Journal of Clinical Investigation* in November, 1990 showed that animals given this Japanese batch of L-tryptophan developed symptoms like those resulting in the human deaths, while pure grade L-tryptophan produced no such symptoms.[6]

The FDA nevertheless refused to allow L-tryptophan back on the market. This policy, noted health writer Gary Null, contrasted sharply with the FDA's treatment of major pharmaceuticals. Tylenol and Contac were withdrawn from the market when deaths resulted from contaminated batches, but they were reintroduced as soon as the problem was identified and corrected. Prozac, acclaimed because it produces fewer unpleasant side effects than prior antidepressants, has been implicated in more than a hundred civil suits and thirty criminal suits involving allegations that it caused violent behavior—including suicide and murder. Yet the FDA has steadfastly declined to withdraw the drug, sales of which are predicted to hit a staggering $2.3 billion by 1994.[7]

Prozac, it turns out, is L-tryptophan's major market competitor. Prozac doesn't actually produce serotonin but is a serotonin "enhancer" that acts by inhibiting a natural process—the reuptake of serotonin by the neurons. Because it affects the body's chemistry in an unbalanced way, it may, unlike L-tryptophan, cause serious side effects.

Diet and exercise

L-tryptophan is now back on the market, but only by prescription; and it is quite expensive. Fortunately, there are other ways of elevating your serotonin levels that don't require drugs or supplements.

One is exercise, which leads to higher brain concentrations of serotonin and norepinephrine, another depression reliever.[9] Running is well known for the "runner's high." Dr. Peat cautions, however, that jogging carries certain risks as you get older, including blood clotting, which can increase the risk of strokes and heart attacks; flat feet; varicose veins; and uterine prolapse.[10] Walking, swimming, and low-impact aerobics are safer alternatives.

Another way to raise brain levels of serotonin is to change your diet. Researchers at MIT found that women who binged on high-carbohydrate foods before menstruation experienced relief of depression, anger, tension, tiredness, and moodiness. These effects were attributed to an elevation in serotonin levels.[11]

On the other hand, you should avoid sugary foods, which can wreak havoc on your blood sugar level. Erratic drops in blood sugar can cause both depression and binging. The best carbohydrates are whole grains—oatmeal and other whole grain cereals, whole grain breads, rice, and potatoes. For the many people who are allergic to wheat, there are several whole grain alternatives to this popular favorite.

Mood-elevating herbs and nutritional supplements

The Oriental explanation for menopausal depression is that it results from stagnation of the liver meridian. When the liver isn't functioning properly, the blood doesn't flow freely and the liver doesn't clean it properly. Hormones aren't broken down well and depression results. When your energy doesn't flow evenly, you stagnate; you feel like a stagnant pool. The Chinese remedy is an herbal formula called *Hsiao Yao Wan*. It stimulates the liver energy to work more actively, relieving the stagnant feeling. Depression typically lifts within a few days. American-made versions have the brand names *Relaxed Wanderer* and *Bupleurum and Peony*. (See Figure 7.)

If depression is also linked to anxiety, palpitations, nightmares, or panic attacks, the heart meridian is usually involved. For an out-of-balance heart meridian, the Chinese have other herbal formulas, including *Anmien Pien*, *Pai Tzu Yang Hsin Wan*, and *Hu Po Yang Xin Dan*.

One of the safest and most effective products now available for relieving stress and giving you a lift is a Bach Flower combination formula called *Rescue Remedy*. Bach Flower remedies were discovered in the nineteenth century by a British physician, Edward Bach, M.D. *Rescue Remedy* has worked well for thousands of people and is currently the single best-selling product at the holistic drugstore where Dr. Walker advises patients on the use of remedies. The recommended dosage is a mere four drops mixed in water, sipped throughout the day; or one drop taken directly under the tongue. There are also thirty-eight individual Bach Flower remedies for specific depression symptoms. Although they require patience, if taken over several months they can be very effective at calming the disposition.

For relieving insomnia, evening primrose oil taken orally at night can be quite effective. Melatonin is another option that has been promoted lately in the media, but Dr. Walker has found it to be more useful for men than women. It is also liable to propel women into hot flashes. This is also true for the stimulant herb Ma Huang and for diet pills, which change the thermogenesis of the body.

Over-the-counter remedies useful for depression, insomnia and related symptoms are listed in Figure 7.

Homeopathic Remedies for Depression
Depression (Extrovert)
Depression (Introvert)
Anti-Depression
Hysteria

Made by
Professional Health
Professional Health
Professional Health
Professional Health

Amino Acid Products for Depression
Catemine
L-Tyrosine
Norival

Tyson
Tyson
Cardiovascular Research

Herbal Formulas for Insomnia
Melatone
VPB
Valerian/Passion Flower
Dormeasan
Valerian Herbal
Zizyphus
Zizyphus
Naturest

Cardiovascular Research
NF Formulas
Eclectic
Bioforce
McZand
McZand
Seven Forests
Nature's Way

Homeopathic Remedies for Insomnia
Insomnia
Quietude
Alpha N.D.
Snoozers

Natra-Bio
Boiron
Boericke & Tafel
Boericke & Tafel

Homeopathic Remedies for Anxiety and Nervousness
Calms
Calms Forte
Nervousness
Insomnia/Anxiety

Hylands
Hylands
Boiron
Dolisos

Herbal Formulas for Anxiety and Nervousness
Alfalco
Rescue Remedy
Ex Stress
Less Stress
Fu-shen 16

Boericke & Tafel
Bach Flowers
Nature's Way
Jade
Seven Forests

Figure 7: Remedies for Depression, Insomnia, and Related Symptoms

III

Nutritional and
Lifestyle Solutions

Chapter Fourteen

Diet, Exercise, and Hormone Balance

Better to hunt in fields, for health unbought,
Than fee the doctor for a nauseous draught.
The wise, for cure, on exercise depend;
God never made his work, for man to mend.
—John Dryden (1631–1700)

Metabolism can slow down at menopause by as much as 25 percent. To avoid putting on weight, you may need to exercise more, eat less, or both. Exercise not only balances your metabolic slowdown but counteracts depression and anxiety and improves glucose control.

In addition to relieving menopausal symptoms, proper diet and exercise are your most natural options for avoiding heart disease, cancer, and osteoporosis. Women following traditional lifestyles in some non-Western cultures are reported not only to have very low incidences of these diseases but to be virtually free of menopausal symptoms.[1]

Diet, estrogen levels, and menopausal complaints

High levels of estrogen, along with imbalances in the other female hormones, have been blamed for many women's complaints, from PMS and menopausal symptoms to abnormal bleeding from the uterus, earlier onset of menstruation, late cessation of menstrual flow at menopause, fibroids of the uterus, and an increased risk of cancer of the uterus.[2] Excess estrogen may come from estrogen overproduction, insufficient levels of progesterone to oppose it, or insufficient estrogen breakdown caused by enzyme deficiency or by diseases of the lower bowel or of the liver. All of these imbalances can be due to nutritional imbalances.

Dietary sources of estrogen that can contribute to estrogen excess include meat from hormone-fed livestock and poultry. Non-dietary sources include cosmetics made with hormones and estrogen replacement therapy that is not opposed by progesterone.

Another nutritional link is with dietary fat. Animal fats inhibit the production of progesterone. They encourage the growth of intestinal bacteria that convert progesterone-opposing estrogen from its inactive to its active form. They are also the raw material for a certain prostaglandin (F2-alpha) that causes the ovaries to decrease progesterone production.[3] Lowering the fat intake will quickly change the levels of estrogen, progesterone, and testosterone in the body. Women eating a typically high-fat American diet have approximately one-third higher levels of estrogen in their blood than women on low-fat vegetarian diets.[4]

Fat is also linked to obesity, which is the most common cause of estrogen overproduction. (Other causes are stress and ovarian cysts.) In obese women, estrogen levels increase when androgens are converted to estrogen. Women who are twenty-five to fifty pounds overweight have a threefold increase in the risk of endometrial hyperplasia, while women who are more than fifty pounds overweight have a ninefold increase in this cancer-disposing condition.[5]

A relatively painless way to lose weight is to replace fat calories with complex carbohydrates—whole grains, rice, and potatoes. These high-fiber foods aid elimination and fill you up more, making you satisfied with fewer calories. They also help fight heart disease and cancer. (See Ellen H. Brown, *With the Grain: Eat More, Weigh Less, Live Longer.*[6])

Dietary fiber can also help keep estrogen levels from going too high. Fiber binds with the deactivated estrogen and moves it through the intestines.[7] Studies show that women on high-fiber, low-fat diets have less PMS, less breast cancer, less premenstrual breast pain, and less trouble with their menstrual periods.[8]

Other studies suggest that the lack of menopausal complaints in women in some non-Western cultures may be due to the high amounts of plant sterols in their diets. Plant sterols are easily converted to human estrogen and progesterone in the body. The difference between getting hormones from pills or hormone-fed meats and getting them from plants is that in the plant form, you're getting only the precursors. Your body can take from these building blocks and make whatever it needs. You don't have to fear pushing your estrogen levels to dangerous heights.[9]

A Finnish study published in the British medical journal *The Lancet* in May, 1992 found that Japanese women, who have few unpleasant postmenopausal symptoms, excrete 1,000 times the amount of phytoestrogens (plant estrogens) as do women in Finland. Soy products high in phytoestrogens are eaten in abundance by the Japanese.[10]

Another study, published in the *British Medical Journal* in 1990, found that menopausal symptoms were significantly reduced in twenty-five women on a diet high in phytoestrogens. Phytoestrogens were furnished in that study in the form of soya flour, red clover sprouts, and linseed or flax seed oil.[11]

Other foods high in plant hormones include yams, papayas, peas, cucumbers, bananas, bee pollen, raw nuts, seeds, sprouts, and certain herbs, including alfalfa, licorice root, red clover, sage, sarsaparilla, and sassafras. Naturopathic doctors who specialize in natural remedies also recommend the following foods to counteract menopausal complaints: raw fruits, fresh fruit and vegetable juices (especially green juices), leafy green vegetables, garlic, figs, dates, cabbage, avocados, grapes, apples, beets, spirulina, chlorella, seaweed, wheat germ, and wheat germ oil.

Citrus fruits, cherries, grapes, hawthorn berry, and red clover are good sources of estrogen-containing bioflavonoids. Bioflavonoids have been found to be effective in controlling hot flashes, anxiety, and irritability, even though they're only a tiny fraction as strong as drugstore estrogen. They also help in strengthening the capillaries and preventing heavy irregular menstrual bleeding.

The oils of seeds and nuts can also help counteract the dry skin, dry hair, and dry vaginal tissues that plague menopausal women. These symptoms can indicate a lack of essential fatty acids (EFAs). (They're "essential" because they can't be made by the body but have to be ingested.) EFAs include two families of fats, omega-3 fatty acids from linolenic acid and omega-6 fatty acids from linoleic acid. Both are found in high concentrations in linseed or flax seed oil. To counteract dry skin, two teaspoons of this oil are recommended daily. The omega-6 fatty acids are also found in seeds and seed oils generally, including safflower, sunflower, corn, sesame seed, and wheat germ oils; while the omega-3 fatty acids are found in walnut, soybean, and fish oils.

Menopausal complaints can also be relieved by reducing or avoiding certain foods, including not only animal fats and red meat but sugar, soft drinks, chocolate, and coffee. Eating large amounts of sugary foods causes sodium and water retention by causing an abrupt increase in insulin, which suppresses ketoacid formation. The sudden rise in blood sugar caused by sugar and caffeine is also followed by a precipitous fall that leads to hypoglycemia and adrenal burn-out.

Diet and cancer

The plant estrogens and progesterones in the soy products relished by the Japanese may help explain another trait of Japanese women: they have unusually low rates of breast cancer. The researchers finding a thousandfold increase in phytoestrogen excretion in these women reported a breast cancer risk that was only about one-fifth that in the United States.[12]

Breast cancer incidence is six times as high in Western countries as in Asian and underdeveloped countries, where the diet centers around vegetables, fish, and grains instead of high-fat animal foods. The risk goes up for women who move from underdeveloped countries to the United States, suggesting an environmental rather than a hereditary cause.[13]

If breast cancer is stimulated by estrogen, why would plant estrogens reduce its incidence? The researchers studying the Japanese suggested that soy phytoestrogens bind to estrogen receptors in place of the body's own estrogen, preventing it from stimulating the growth

114

of cancer cells. That makes phytoestrogens a much safer and cheaper option than anti-cancer drugs like tamoxifen, which also prevents estrogen from stimulating cancer growth but in a less natural way that can produce unwanted side effects.[14]

Many other cancer anti-promoters (substances that discourage tumor formation) are provided by plant foods. They include nutritional antioxidants, particularly vitamins A, C, and E, found in large quantities in fruits and vegetables; fiber, found only in plants; cruciferous vegetables (broccoli, cabbage, cauliflower); beans and seeds.[15]

Other anti-cancer features of traditional non-Western diets are that they're low in fat, low in protein, and low in calories. High intakes of these dietary components are all linked to high estrogen levels, which are linked, in turn, to high rates of the hormone-dependent cancers of the breast, ovary, testis, prostate and uterus.[16] These cancers occur ten times as frequently in the United States as in Japan, and five times as frequently as in India and Central Europe.[17]

Breast cancer, the leading hormone-dependent cancer in women, is highly correlated both with estrogen levels and with the consumption of meat and animal fat.[18] Vegetarian Seventh Day Adventist women, who have a low incidence of breast cancer, excrete greater amounts of this hormone than meat-eating women and have lower levels of it in their blood.[19] Studies also suggest a link between breast cancer and dietary fat of all types, but one problem with the theory is that fat intake in this country hasn't increased in tandem with breast cancer incidence. New studies suggest the critical factor may be not the fat itself but the fat-soluble pollutants it carries. Researchers writing in *Archives of Environmental Health* in April, 1992, found that the tissues of women with breast cancer had concentrations of certain hydrocarbon-based pesticides and polychlorinated biphenyls (PCBs) that were 50 to 60 percent higher than normal.[20] These environmental pollutants are soluble in animal fat and concentrate at the top of the food chain, or in human tissue. This means eating high-fat foods increases your exposure to various cancer-causing chemicals.

In the United States and England, particularly high correlations have been found between breast cancer incidence and milk consumption.[21] Hormonal substances used as growth promoters can also be detected in meat. This may explain why in Japan, where milk is not a major item in the diet, breast cancer incidence is 8.5 times as high among women who eat meat daily as among those who do not.[22]

Dietary supplements you can take to help ward off cancer include vitamins A, C, and E, evening primrose oil and black currant seed oil. (See Chapter Fifteen.) Another option is the amino acid L-arginine, which has been shown to effectively prevent cancer and shrink tumors in animals and to bolster the immune system in humans. L-arginine can also help rejuvenate the body, slim it down, and tone it up.[23]

Diet and bone loss

Women in some non-Western cultures manage to escape not only cancer but the increased rate of hip fractures experienced by Western women after menopause. Oddly, their calcium intakes tend to be below those of American women.[24] If a high calcium intake isn't the secret to good bones, what is? Other proposed answers are low intakes of protein, meat, and phosphorus; a high intake of potassium; and regular exercise.

A too-high protein intake has been shown to leach calcium from the bones.[25] A too-low protein intake is also hazardous, however, because protein is necessary for the liver to detoxify estrogen.[26] For bone loss, meat rather than protein may be the critical variable. Vegetarian Seventh Day Adventists, who avoid meat for religious reasons, lose bone at only about half the rate of matched meat-eating women.[27]

Meat is high not only in protein but in phosphorus, which has also been linked to bone loss. Each phosphorus atom in the bloodstream must be accompanied by a calcium atom. The calcium pulled out of the blood to pair up with this phosphorus is replaced with calcium from the bones. Phosphorus is also antagonistic to potassium, a mineral found in the unprocessed vegetables, fruits, and whole grains abundant in traditional non-Western diets. Calcium-and potassium-robbing phosphorus is supplied in the Western diet not only by meat but by worse offenders, carbonated soft drinks.

Exercise is another variable. Walking is something Western women do occasionally for health. For many women in non-Western countries, walking is transportation. It's how they get to work and how they get their water from the river or communal tap, gliding gracefully over long distances with heavy jugs balanced on their heads. This is "weight-bearing exercise" in its original form.

Clinical studies show that weight-bearing exercise like brisk walking, jogging, low impact aerobics, and trampoline-jumping improves bone density and prevents osteoporosis. It also forestalls cardiovascular disease and prevents or relieves obesity, muscle weakness, and depression. Studies also show, fortunately, that you don't have to train like an Olympic athlete to improve cardiovascular fitness. Thirty minutes three times a week seem to be enough.[28]

Diet and heart disease

High blood levels of estrogen have been linked to both cancer and heart disease.[29] The elevated levels of blood pressure and serum cholesterol that are major risk factors for heart disease and stroke are favorite targets of the drug industry; but the drug approach carries its own risks and has not been proven to extend life. (See Chapter 16.) Fortunately, most people can lower both their serum cholesterol and blood pressure levels without drugs, merely by changing their diets. The dietary approach can be as effective as drugs without unwanted side effects. More important, for people whose risk factors have been lowered in this way, life expectancy has actually increased.[30]

In a study reported in the *New England Journal of Medicine* in 1987, adding only a single serving of fruit or vegetables to the daily diet was found to lower the risk of stroke by a full 40 percent, about the same benefit as a full course of antihypertensive drugs and without the side effects. Stroke deaths varied inversely with the intake of potassium, a mineral that is prevalent in unprocessed plant foods. As potassium went up, deaths from stroke went down.[31]

Interestingly, the intake of sodium (from salt), the dietary variable most often associated with high blood pressure, wasn't significantly related to stroke deaths. It is the *ratio* of sodium to potassium that's important. Whole cereals, all fruits, and most vegetables contain from ten to one hundred times as much potassium as sodium.

However, the modern diet contains more sodium than potassium, mainly because potassium is removed and sodium added during processing and cooking. (See Figure 8.)

Serum cholesterol can also be lowered by a high-fiber diet centered around unprocessed plant foods. Insoluble fiber, the kind in wheat bran, increases stool bulk and promotes bowel function, but the type of fiber that seems to be best for lowering serum cholesterol is the soluble fiber found in fruits, vegetables, and oat bran. Insoluble fibers remain coarse and gritty in water, while soluble fibers dissolve to form a gel which traps cholesterol-rich bile acids that would otherwise have been recycled. When they're trapped and eliminated, the body has to use up other cholesterol to make more bile acids, and serum cholesterol is reduced.[32]

Soluble fiber is also found in bulk laxatives containing psyllium, including Metamucil, Konsyl, and Modane Bulk. In a 1988 study, volunteers with an average serum cholesterol level of 250 mg/dl were given a teaspoonful of Metamucil three times a day. After eight weeks, their cholesterol levels had dropped an average of 35 mg/dl, or 14 percent. This result was about as good as with the riskier bile-acid resin drugs Questran and Colestin.

In fact, the soluble fiber in psyllium works in much the same way as these drugs. It binds bile acids in the intestines and prevents them from being reabsorbed. Psyllium has several advantages over drugs—it's easier to swallow, side effects are limited to occasional mild stomach cramps and gas, and it's substantially cheaper.[33]

Common edible plant fibers, including the pectin found in apples and other fruits and vegetables, lower cholesterol in the same way. In combination with calcium, pectin binds readily to bile acids, rendering them useless as digestive enzymes. The liver senses there is a shortage of bile acid and compensates by extracting cholesterol molecules from the blood. These molecules are then modified into bile molecules. The result is a drop in serum cholesterol.[34]

It is important not merely to reduce the fat in your diet but to substitute high-fiber plant foods in its place. An Indian study reported in 1992 found that a diet stressing fruits, grains, nuts, fish, and vegetables protects the heart better than merely cutting back on high-

	[mg/100g]	
	Sodium	Potassium
Flour, wholemeal	3	360
White bread	540	100
Rice, polished	6	110
Rice, boiled	2	38
Beef, uncooked	55	280
Beef, corned	950	140
Haddock, uncooked	120	300
Haddock, smoked	790	190
Cabbage, uncooked	7	390
Cabbage, boiled	4	160
Peas, uncooked	1	340
Peas, canned	230	130
Pears, uncooked	2	130
Pears, canned	1	90

**Figure 8. Sodium and Potassium Contents
of Some Common Foods — Processed vs. Unprocessed**

fat meats and dairy products. The number of prior heart attack victims who suffered second heart attacks or sudden death on this diet
was only half of those on a low-fat diet.[35]

To sum up, a diet centered around whole, unprocessed plant foods
can lower your blood pressure, lower your serum cholesterol, protect
you against cancer, reduce your weight, and help replace and balance
your lost ovarian hormones.

Chapter Fifteen

Support from Nutritional Supplements

Twenty years from now, physicians may well be prescribing
custom-tailored cocktails that will protect the elderly from
degenerative damage, help them stay physically active and
generally improve the quality of their lives.

—Daniel Rudman, Veterans Affairs
Medical Center, Milwaukee[1]

Ideally, we would get sufficient vitamins, minerals, and amino acids
from our food. But pesticides and other chemical pollutants in our
environment have diminished the value of our food supply, and years
of dietary abuse have exhausted our natural reserves. Replenishing
these deficiencies is likely to require nutritional supplements. We'll
start with an overview of useful supplements, then focus on the more
interesting ones in detail.

Nutrients important for maintaining hormone balance and adequate hormone synthesis include the following:

Anti-stress vitamins involved in progesterone production include
vitamin A, *vitamin C*, *panthothenic acid*, and *vitamin E*. Vitamin E and
panthothenic acid can also help reduce hot flashes.

Iodine, *manganese* and *cobalt* are needed by the thyroid.[2]

Nutrients that are depleted by excess estrogen include *folic acid*,
zinc, and *vitamin B6*. Sufficient vitamin B6 is required for the liver
to deactivate estrogen, and sufficient *vitamin B2* and *magnesium* are
required to activate the B6. Magnesium also opposes estrogen and

121

calcium in the clotting system. *B vitamins* generally (along with sufficient protein) are needed to regulate the estrogen level.

Estrogen production and prostaglandin synthesis can be maintained, and PMS symptoms can be relieved, with *evening primrose oil, black currant oil,* or *borage.*

Calcium, magnesium, and *vitamin D* are necessary to maintain the bones. Calcium and magnesium also help relieve nervousness and irritability.

The digestive ailments that arise when the acid output of the stomach drops off with age can be relieved with *acidophilus* or with *pancreatic enzymes* (although the FDA may soon be removing the latter from the market). *Chromium* helps regulate blood sugar levels and plays a vital role in the metabolism of sugar, protein, and fat. The most absorbable form available is *chromium picolinate.* Taken twice daily, at 10 AM and 2 PM, it can help you maintain an even blood sugar level throughout the day, quelling the urge to nibble.

Bovine glandular extracts help augment uterine and ovarian function. If the uterus is weak, you can supplement either with natural progesterone or with *Utrophin* to stimulate its production. If the ovaries are weak, you can supplement either with estrogen or with *Ovex* to stimulate its production. In women who still have their ovaries, progesterone levels may also be raised by *Ovatrophin,* made from bovine corpus luteum (the part of the cow ovary that contains progesterone).

Some over-the-counter nutritional products beneficial for menopausal and premenstrual problems are listed in Figure 9.

Vitamin E

Medical studies have shown Vitamin E to be quite effective in reducing hot flashes.[3] Hormone researcher Ray Peat says the data adds support to the theory that hot flashes are due to a progesterone deficiency rather than an estrogen deficiency. Vitamin E is antagonistic in many ways to estrogen and has been called the "anti-estrogenic vitamin." Estrogen seems to increase the body's need for vitamin E.[4]

Vitamin E is also useful for relieving other menopausal complaints, including breast tenderness and vaginal dryness. It is involved in progesterone synthesis and helps preserve ATP, a source of biologi-

Vitamins for Menopause	Made by*
Gynovite	Optimox
Change of Life	Ethical Nutrients
Fem Estro	Metagenics
Fem Utero	Metagenics
Fem FBS	Metagenics
Vitamins for PMS	
Maxovite	Tyson
Optivite	Optimox
Vita Gyn	Eclectic
Fem PMS	Metagenics
Fem UBF	Metagenics
Support for the Bones	
Urticalcin	Bioforce
Cal Apatite	Metagenics
Osteomatria	Probiologics
Osteo-Novum	Cardiovascular Research
For Prostaglandin Synthesis	
Evening Primrose Oil	Nature's Way and others
Black Currant Seed Oil	Eclectic and others
Glandular Extracts	
Ovex	Standard Process
Ovatrophin	Standard Process
Utrophin	Standard Process
	* See the Appendix.

Figure 9: Nutritional Support for Hormone-Related Problems

cal energy and a tissue relaxant. (The closely related *coenzyme Q10* has similar properties and is another energy booster.)

When buying vitamin E, look for the natural product (d-alpha tocopherol or d-alpha tocopheryl), which is absorbed better from the digestive system and retained in the body longer than synthetic vitamin E (dl-alpha tocopherol or dl-alpha tocopheryl).[5] Vitamin E is also absorbed better when taken with meals than on an empty stomach. It should not be taken with iron supplements, which destroy it.

Iron-rich foods like raisins and spinach, on the other hand, can be eaten without harm to the vitamin E.

Vitamin E is one of those vitamins you can get too much of, but for hot flashes, 400 to 600 international units (IU) can safely be taken daily without a prescription.[6] For quelling intractable hot flashes, some physicians recommend up to 1600 IU per day.[7] If you experience blurred vision, you should stop taking the vitamin.

If you're not struggling with hot flashes, lower doses are sufficient. In one study, taking 150 IU of vitamin E daily increased progesterone levels, while higher doses, ranging from 300 to 600 IU, actually lowered progesterone levels.[8] For protecting your heart, a mere 100 IU daily appears to be enough. In two studies reported in 1992 involving more than 130,000 people, women who took at least 100 IU per day of vitamin E for two or more years reduced their risk of heart disease by 26 percent, and men on the same regimen reduced their risk by 46 percent. People who took megadoses of vitamin E had no greater reduction in risk than those who took 100 IU daily.[9]

Iron

Some studies have found that iron can relieve heavy menstrual bleeding, but the supplement is controversial. Recent studies link too much iron to an increased risk of heart disease. A Finnish study that followed 1,931 men for five years found that men with high blood iron levels faced more than double the risk of heart attack. The researchers went so far as to put elevated iron as the second largest risk factor for heart disease, preceded only by smoking.[10] Until menopause, women have a significantly lower incidence of heart disease than men. This has normally been ascribed to the protective effects of estrogen, but some scientists now wonder if a woman's lower iron levels may not also be a factor. Menstruation depletes the body's iron stores through blood loss.[11]

Calcium, magnesium, and bone loss

Calcium is a popular supplement among women concerned with bone loss. However, calcium is antagonistic to magnesium, and both are critical nutrients. Excess calcium causes magnesium depletion, which can lead to irritability, blood clots, vascular spasms, and angina pectoris.[12]

Magnesium is also essential for moving calcium out of the bloodstream and into the skeleton. Without it, the calcium you eat may never make it to your bones. Calcium is a heavy metal. If it's not assimilated well, it may settle out of your blood and contribute to kidney stones and impaired kidney function, or to soft tissue calcification and arthritis. Calcium can also bind to other material in the intestines and cause constipation. Magnesium has the opposite effect on elimination.[13]

Guy E. Abraham, M.D., a research gynecologist in Torrance, California, increased bone density in postmenopausal women by 11 percent in one year, by *lowering* their calcium intake to 500 milligrams (mg) per day and *increasing* their magnesium intake to 600-1000 mg per day. He based the dose of magnesium on bowel tolerance: diarrhea was the limiting factor.

Dr. Abraham's results were significantly better than in studies involving calcium alone. In fact few studies have shown that calcium supplements have any effect on bone density.[14] In those that have, the calcium sources were particularly bioavailable (available for use by the body). Even with the more bioavailable calcium sources, however, bone density gains have not compared to the 11 percent gains with magnesium supplements or the 15 to 30 percent gains with natural progesterone.[15]

One highly bioavailable calcium source, little known in the United States but widely used in Europe, is *microcrystalline hydroxyapatite compound* (MCHC). MCHC is the organic protein calcium matrix found in the raw young bones of cattle and sheep raised on insecticide-and pesticide-free pastures. It differs from bone meal, which also comes from bone, in that it's not heated in the reduction process or washed with chemical solvents. In two recent studies comparing MCHC with calcium gluconate and a placebo in the treatment of postmenopausal osteoporosis, only the MCHC groups experienced a significant increase in cortical bone.[16]

A cheaper option that can also put bone back on is *calcium citrate*. Calcium absorption from calcium citrate is as much as four times as great as that from calcium carbonate; and absorption from a combination chelate called *calcium citrate-malate* (CCM) is better yet.[17]

Calcium carbonate is the kind of calcium found in antacid lozenges like Tums, often recommended as a cheap calcium source. However, the purpose of an antacid is to neutralize stomach acid, and when stomach acid is neutralized, the absorption of calcium and other nutrients is impaired.

Whatever the source, if you are taking calcium, you should take magnesium in a dosage high enough to counterbalance it. Magnesium is abundant in whole grains, beans, nuts, seeds, and vegetables. Fertilizers reduce its content in the soil, while sugar and alcohol increase its excretion through the urine. The RDA for magnesium is only 350 mg for women of all ages. However, Dr. Mildred Seelig, Executive President of the American College of Nutrition, suggests that older people eating a good diet can benefit from magnesium supplements of 700-800 mg per day. Dr. Peat recommends 1000 mg per day.[18]

Calcium, magnesium, and PMS

Some research suggests that calcium may be useful in the treatment of PMS. A 1991 USDA study found that women with PMS had lower blood calcium levels than other women. Calcium levels were particularly low during their PMS symptoms. Symptoms were noticeably relieved in nine out of ten women when calcium intake was boosted to 1300 mg per day.[19] A 1989 study reached the same result using 1000 mg of calcium from calcium carbonate, with 73 percent of thirty-three women reporting fewer symptoms during calcium treatment.[20]

Another study, however, showed that women with the most common type of PMS (characterized by anxiety, irritability, and mood swings) ate five times the amount of dairy products as women not suffering from the condition. Oddly, dairy products are high in calcium. The PMS sufferers also ate three times the amount of refined sugar as other women.[21]

The ill effects of sugar are easiest to explain. Sugar increases the excretion of magnesium and impairs estrogen deactivation by the liver. The ill effects of dairy products could also involve magnesium.

126

Dairy products contain nine times as much calcium as magnesium, so ingesting them in large quantities can upset your calcium/magnesium balance. Magnesium is helpful in battling PMS because it helps the body use B vitamins and inactivate excess estrogen.[22] It also helps with painful periods. A recent study found that in women with this problem, magnesium significantly reduced lower abdominal and back pain.[23]

Dairy products have other drawbacks besides upsetting magnesium balance. They are high in protein, which pulls calcium from the bones; and many people have lost the ability to properly digest and metabolize them. Milk allergy is one of the commonest food allergies. Fortunately, there are non-dairy dietary sources of calcium that are just as good as milk. Cows get calcium directly from the plants that get it from the soil. High-calcium foods are listed in Figure 10 in order of calories per 300 milligrams of calcium.[24]

Other nutritional supplements shown to relieve PMS symptoms include vitamin B6, vitamin E, and essential fatty acids. Avoidance of caffeine and allergenic foods can also help.[25]

Evening primrose oil and black currant oil

These supplements are useful for the treatment of hot flashes and the production of estrogen.[26] They are also among the few readily available sources of gamma-linolenic acid (GLA), essential for making the prostaglandin that counters cramps and painful menstruation.

Prostaglandins are hormone-like chemical substances that perform a variety of opposing functions. Some stimulate the contraction of smooth muscle tissue, including the contractions that expel babies and menstrual blood. The "bad" prostaglandin called PGE2 is thought to be responsible for cramps and painful menstruation. It has also been blamed for the depression, fluid retention, and breast pain and tenderness that characterize PMS, although an alternative theory blames the hormone prolactin.[27]

Harmful prostaglandins can be suppressed by drugs called prostaglandin inhibitors, but the drugs themselves may have harmful side effects. The other option is to increase blood levels of the "good" prostaglandin PGE1, which tempers the bad effects of both

Food	Calcium (mgs)	Calories
1 cup cooked bok choy	300	25
1 cup cooked collards	300	60
1¼ cups other greens, cooked	300	60
2 cups cooked broccoli	300	80
1 cup skim milk	300	90
½ cup plain low-fat yogurt	300	95
1 cup buttermilk	300	100
2½ tablespoons blackstrap molasses	300	110
1/4 cup grated Parmesan cheese	300	115
1 cup low-fat milk	300	120
1½ ounces cheddar, Swiss or American cheese	300	150
1 cup whole milk	300	150
8 ounces tofu	300	150
½ cup part skim milk ricotta	300	170
3½ ounce can sardines drained	300	200
3½ ounce can sardines in sauce	300	230
1 cup fruit flavored yogurt	300	200–280
5 ounces canned salmon	300	235
1½ cups ice milk	300	325
2 cups low-fat cottage cheese	300	410
7 corn tortillas	300	420
1¼ cups ice cream	300	450–1000

Figure 10. High-Calcium Low-Calorie Foods

PGE2 and prolactin. PGE1 is converted from linoleic acid (found in safflower, sunflower, corn, sesame, flax, soybean, and pumpkin seed oils), while PGE2 is converted from arachidonic acid (found in meat, eggs, and dairy products).

In theory, you should be able to augment your PGE1 by increasing your intake of the linoleic acid from which it is made. But linoleic acid is two stages away from PGE1, and many people don't convert it well. The fragile step involves a delicate enzyme that can be blocked by a number of factors common to modern-day diets and lifestyles. They include excess saturated fat (found in animal fats, coconut oil, and palm kernel oil), trans fatty acids (found in margarine, vegetable shortening, pastries, chips, and fries), oxidizing chemicals (including indoor pollutants and cigarette smoke), environmental pollutants, ionizing radiation, alcohol, cortisone, high cholesterol levels, refined sugar and flour, aspirin (a drug unsuspecting sufferers are liable to take to *relieve* their premenstrual headaches), and stress (which causes the adrenal glands to release epinephrine).[28]

If you can't avoid these enzyme inhibitors, you can avoid the enzyme stage altogether by ingesting GLA directly. The problem is that GLA is available in only a few natural substances. One of them is human breast milk, suggesting its importance in human nutrition and breast function. Unfortunately, GLA is not available in cow's milk.[29] The most accessible food sources are *evening primrose oil, black currant oil, borage oil, spirulina,* and *chlorella.*

Evening primrose oil, a traditional North American Indian remedy, is the GLA source that has been most often studied. In one series of four studies, modest amounts of evening primrose oil substantially improved PMS symptoms even in stubborn cases that responded to nothing else. Three of these studies were double-blind and placebo-controlled. Evening primrose oil also reversed benign breast disease, an objective result not subject to the placebo effect.[30] In fact it proved to be so safe and effective for this purpose that some doctors in England now use it as the treatment of first choice in this painful condition.[31]

Evening primrose oil has also been shown to lower blood pressure, lower serum cholesterol, decrease the amount of insulin required by diabetics, and aid in weight loss by increasing fat metabolism. Cofactors in the body's conversion of GLA to PGE1 that should accompany its intake are zinc and vitamins C, B3, and B6.[32]

A cheaper but less studied GLA source is black currant seed oil. Some research suggests its GLA may not be converted to PGEl as efficiently,[33] but it has the advantage that it contains the beneficial omega-3 fatty acids along with the omega-6 fatty acids and GLA. Omega-3 and omega-6 fatty acids must be eaten in balanced quantities for proper prostaglandin formation; but American omega-3 intake has decreased by nearly 80 percent over the last century, throwing the proportions out of balance.[34]

Omega-3 and omega-6 fatty acids both help protect against a number of diseases, including heart disease, PMS, cancer, and rheumatoid arthritis. In a 1987 study from the Glasgow Royal Infirmary in Scotland, rheumatoid arthritis patients treated with either omega-3 or omega-6 fatty acids were so much improved that 60 percent were able to stop their normal anti-arthritis medications. Patients receiving both EFAs together showed even greater improvement. Other researchers have studied the optimal ratio of omega-3 to omega-6 fatty acids in the diet. They suggest an ideal ratio of about one to five, which happens to be the ratio found in black currant oil.[35]

Dr. Lynne Walker uses black currant oil to reduce inflammation. She has found it can work as well on asthma and other breathing problems as steroids like prednisone, without the devastating side effects of steroids. Inflammation is produced by PGE2 and reduced by PGE1.

PGE1 (which is converted from the GLA in evening primrose oil and black currant oil) also has other beneficial functions. It prevents the blood platelet aggregation that causes heart attacks and strokes, opens up blood vessels and improves circulation, helps the kidneys remove fluid from the body, slows down cholesterol production, controls arthritis, improves nerve function and gives a sense of well-being, regulates calcium metabolism, and aids the immune system.[36] Research also suggests that GLA inhibits the development of cancer.[37]

Chapter Sixteen

Saying No to Drugs

The pharmaceuticals industry Code of Ethics does not allow the production of any product unless merely pronouncing its chemical name in front of laboratory rats causes at least a third of them to die.

—Humor writer Dave Barry[1]

Hormone synthesis can fail not only from lack of nutrients but from antagonistic substances that counteract them, including drugs. Synthetic pharmaceuticals can substantially alter the biological impact and metabolism of the steroid hormones, including estrogen and progesterone.[2] All drugs throw your system off to some extent, and if they can be avoided, they should be. We wrote about this in an earlier book, *The Informed Consumer's Pharmacy.*[3]

Some drugs are specifically intended to suppress hormone production. One is tamoxifen, discussed in Chapter Five. Another is Lupron (leuprolide acetate), a drug given to induce menopause. It is currently popular for conditions that tend to improve after menopause, like fibroid tumors and endometriosis. While it may successfully eliminate the pain of endometriosis, its cost is premature menopause, which is particularly problematic in these cases because the drug tends to be given to women who are still young. Other problems are that it induces hot flashes; women who take it seem to age overnight; and it can cause bone pain, weakness, and numbness in the lower limbs during the first few weeks of treatment.[4]

Other drugs intended to suppress hormone production are used for treating cancer. Antiestrogen therapy with tamoxifen works (when it does, which is about one-third of the time) by preventing estrogen from stimulating the growth of cancer cells. The same mechanism may, in fact, underlie all drugs that work against breast cancer: they damage the ovaries, preventing them from producing estrogen.[5] Hormone balance can also be altered by steroids (estrogens, androgens, progestins, and adrenal corticosteroids). Adrenal steroid hormones, including prednisone and dexamethasone, inhibit cell division and are effective against many cancers; but they also have many serious side effects. This whole class of drugs alters hormone balance, the result we're trying to avoid. Antiestrogen medications like tamoxifen produce menopausal symptoms, including atrophic vaginitis; and this happens even in young premenopausal women.[6]

Yet these drugs are safer than the cytotoxic chemotherapy that works by blocking the division of cells—normal as well as cancerous ones. Half of all cancer patients are now being subjected to these havoc-wreaking drugs, but their effectiveness is increasingly being called into question.[7] There are safer, more natural treatments that are effective against cancer. Most aren't available in the United States, but they are available in Europe and Mexico, where manufacturers of herbal and natural medicines are not required to invest millions in research before marketing their products, encouraging the development and promotion of low-profit, unpatentable traditional remedies.[8]

Drugs that are less dangerous but can still throw your system out of balance include diuretics, or water pills. Both estrogens and progestins increase the uptake of sodium and water by cells, causing water retention and bloating. Diuretics are often recommended to relieve this condition in both PMS sufferers and women on HRT.[9] However, the drugs work by forcing the kidneys to release body fluid; and with the excess water go important minerals and chemicals, throwing off electrolyte and mineral balance. That's why most diuretics are prescription drugs. In fact PMS is the *only* condition for which their over-the-counter use is approved, and that's only because the pills are intended for use only a few days each month. Before you resort

Saying No to Drugs

to them, try drinking less and avoiding salt and salt-rich foods that cause you to retain water. Natural progesterone can eliminate water retention and bloating without side effects, and so can the amino acid L-arginine and certain herbs. Instead of releasing fluid prematurely from the kidneys, they put the whole system back in balance, causing the release of built-up fluid at the cellular level all over the body.

Other drugs are hard on the bones. Among the worst are diuretics like Lasix, given for high blood pressure; and corticosteroids, which have a molecular configuration so like progesterone that the receptor sites get confused, causing advancing osteoporosis. Excess thyroid also destroys bone, by stimulating the osteoclasts to tear it down.[10] Other harmful drugs are antibiotics. They kill off the colon bacteria that make vitamin K, which is involved in bone formation and osteoporosis prevention.[11]

With any drugs, you run the risk of unwanted side effects. In May of 1990, the General Accounting Office, an investigative arm of Congress, released a report stating that more than half the new drugs approved by the FDA for marketing had severe or fatal side effects not found in testing, or not reported until years after the drugs had been in widespread use. The GAO reviewed all the drugs approved for marketing from 1976 to 1985 that were actually sold for a substantial period. Of these drugs—198 in all—102 were found to have side effects serious enough to warrant either withdrawal from the market or major labeling changes.[12]

Even over-the-counter drugs, considered innocuous because they're available without a prescription, can throw your system out of balance and should be avoided when possible. Antacids can affect the absorption of other drugs and nutrients. They can also affect bone mineral metabolism, weakening the bones. Aspirin can cause allergic reactions, irritation and bleeding in the stomach, and anemia through imperceptible iron loss from this bleeding. It can also alter blood coagulation time and lower body temperature. Many drugs inhibit bowel function, leading to chronic constipation. This, in turn, leads to chronic laxative use. The result can be abnormally low blood potassium levels and other electrolyte imbalances.

As we get older, we're likely to take more drugs; but that's also when we're more likely to suffer adverse drug reactions and interactions. Our drug clearance time, the time it takes for medication to pass through the system, gets longer. Kidney function gets worse, and so does blood flow to the liver. Body water decreases and body fat increases. That means water-soluble drugs become more concentrated, and fat-soluble drugs stay around longer and accumulate in the tissues. Moreover, the older we get, the longer our bodies will have been accumulating these drugs. Sedatives and hypnotics can linger in the brain and cause confusion. Drug doses that have been tested on younger people can easily sedate the older person's brain or drop her blood pressure and cause dizziness and fainting.

Drugs that cause dizziness, sedation, and fuzzy thinking can also be responsible for the falls that produce the fractures ERT is recommended to prevent. In one study, older people were found to be about twice as likely to suffer hip fractures if they were taking tranquilizers with long half-lives, like flurazepam (Dalmane); tricyclic antidepressants, including amitriptyline (Elavil), doxepin (Sinequan), and imipramine (Tofranil); or antipsychotics, including thioridazine (Mellaril), haloperidol (Haldol), and chlorpromazine (Thorazine).[14] Diuretic drugs can contribute to hip fractures even if they don't make elderly women dizzy, by necessitating bathroom visits in the middle of the night.

Many of these drugs also impair sexual performance. Antidepressants like Elavil, anti-anxiety preparations like diazepam (Valium) and alprazolam (Xanax), blood pressure medications, and many other pharmaceuticals can decrease sex drive and inhibit orgasm.[15]

But do we dare not take the drugs recommended by our doctors? Jane Brody tells the story of one woman who had the temerity to try it, probably because she was a doctor herself. Dr. Mary Calderone, a woman in her eighties, had been debilitated by extreme sleepiness, loss of balance, loss of memory, weakness, trouble concentrating, depression, and tiredness. Dizziness and instability caused her to take several serious falls. Her doctors said her symptoms were normal for her age, but Dr. Calderone wasn't willing to accept this explanation. She decided to abandon her drugs. The major offender in her case turned out to be the antidepressant Elavil. She'd been taking it in small doses for years to help her get to sleep. When she quit, she got back her energy, her memory, her balance and her ability to think clearly.[16]

That's fine for antidepressants, but what about drugs for lowering blood pressure and serum cholesterol? Wouldn't abandoning them dangerously increase the risk of heart disease and stroke?

Serious damage could indeed be done by stopping some of these drugs suddenly. But weaning from them gradually—under the watchful eye of the licensed practitioner of your choice—while lowering blood pressure or serum cholesterol by more natural means, could improve not only your sense of well-being but your actual chances of survival.

More than sixty million Americans have high blood pressure, and close to half the population over sixty is treated for it. Yet seventy-five percent of these sixty million victims have only "mild" hypertension, and drug treatment for people in this category hasn't been proved to significantly increase survival. Drug therapy became standard treatment before there was reliable evidence of its benefits, and the matter still remains in doubt.[17] Similarly, lowering serum cholesterol with drugs has not been shown in clinical studies to extend life.[18] We saw in Chapter Fourteen that blood pressure and serum cholesterol can be lowered safely through dietary modification and exercise; and when they are lowered in this way, life expectancy is actually increased.

Natural progesterone is another option for lowering blood pressure, especially for women on estrogen. The cellular sodium and water retention caused by estrogen and synthetic progestins can produce not only bloating but a rise in blood pressure. Drug treatment for hypertension can often be avoided in these cases by discontinuing prescription hormones, eliminating sodium-rich processed foods from the diet, and supplementing with natural progesterone.[19] In placebo-controlled studies, natural progesterone has significantly reduced hypertension in both men and women without the use of other antihypertensive drugs.[20]

For virtually every condition that can be treated with drugs, safe natural alternatives are provided by Oriental, herbal, and homeopathic medicine. Many good reference works are available, including Beinfeld's *Between Heaven and Earth: A Guide to Chinese Medicine*, Balch's *Prescription for Nutritional Healing*, and Wiener's *Complete Book of Homeopathy*.[21]

Chapter Seventeen

Longevity

"You are old, Father William," the young man said,
"And your hair has become very white;
"And yet you incessantly stand on your head—
"Do you think, at your age, it is right?"
—*Alice in Wonderland*

Not only are menopausal complaints a disease of civilization; menopause itself might be characterized as one. Animals don't go through it, and the average woman may not have either until recently. In the days of the Roman Empire, life expectancy for a woman was only around twenty-three years. By the fourteenth century, this figure had risen to about thirty-three years; but even at the turn of the twentieth century, female life expectancy was up to only forty-eight years—a couple of years *before* the average modern-day woman can expect to hit menopause. True, these figures averaged in childhood deaths, which were far more common in the past than today. But it is still probably safe to say that for most of recorded history, the majority of women were menstruating for the majority of their adult lives.

Today we can expect to live into our eighties or nineties. If we do, we'll be spending nearly as many years without our premenopausal hormones as with them. "Not too long ago," wrote Dr. Wilson in *Feminine Forever*, "certainly within my own memory—a woman of forty was regarded as being beyond the most significant years of her

ct, the new medical possibilities double a woman's emo-
n."[1]

to Dr. Jiang Fu Jiang, a Chinese medical doctor who teaches at Emperor's College in Los Angeles, if our bodies were kept in perfect balance we could continue menstruating to the end of even a long life. This thought may not appeal to Western women, but menstruation is considered a beneficial cleansing by the Chinese; and an article in the September 1993 issue of the *Quarterly Review of Biology* supports the theory. Evolutionary biologist Margie Profet of the University of California at Berkeley proposes that menstruation is an aggressive way of protecting both mother and fetus from microbes carried into the uterus by penetrating sperm.[2] On that theory, the process should be preserved as long as possible; and in Oriental medicine, the keys to preserving it are certain traditional herbal formulas and acupuncture.

Indian Yogis postulate using the body's own hormones for healing. "The practice of Yoga teaches you how to use your own hormones and your own endocrine glands while they are in the living state of your body," says Indian doctor Rammurti Mishra, M.D. "Yoga psychology teaches you how to heal yourself by your own hormones, how to tranquilize your mind by your own power of thought, how to extract your own hormones from your glands, how to prepare them to heal your mental and physical diseases, and how to develop your body, senses and the mind by them."[3] (For more about yoga, see Chapter Eighteen.)

The theory is appealing, but mastering the skill could take some time. In the meantime, a number of natural substances can help preserve hormone balance, increase longevity, and enhance your sense of youth. Though these sound like snake oil claims, thousands of people regularly use natural remedies for this purpose in Europe, the Far East, and the United States, and testimonials abound that they work. Popular options include *ginseng, Siberian ginseng, Eight Flavor Tea, Gerovital (GH3)*, and the brain-clearing leaf extract *Gingko biloba*.

Coenzyme Q10 is taken daily by over fifteen million Japanese and ranks in sales with Japan's top five drugs. Recent research indicates it's a powerful antioxidant that protects the heart. It resembles vitamin E and is crucial in immunity and the aging process; and body stores decline with age, indicating the need for supplements. Though popular with the Japanese, coenzyme Q10 was actually discovered in the United States in 1957. The reason it is still not a "household nutrient" in the West, according to researcher Dr. Karl Folkers, has more to do with the lack of protected marketing positions than with its safety or how well it works.[5]

Another youth-extender that we've discussed at length is *natural progesterone*. John Lee, M.D., recommends it for any postmenopausal woman interested in preserving her bones. That could mean thirty or forty years of hormone use; but Dr. Lee maintains, "Once you're on it, you might as well stay on it, because it has only healthy benefits. Studies show that if people are on a successful osteoporosis treatment and then quit, the bones quickly lose their bone density."

Natural progesterone also helps maintain brain function, glucose metabolism, sodium regulation, thyroid hormone function, and a healthy uterine lining. It can reverse the chemical changes that occur in collagen, promoting smooth and youthful skin. It aids digestion and helps maintain the thymus.[6]

A properly functioning immune system is, in fact, vital to longevity. The immune system is what protects our bodies from their enemies: bacteria, viruses, tumors, and atherosclerotic plaques. The diseases most likely to kill us can all be held at bay by a properly functioning immune system. Conversely, death results when the immune system has deteriorated so much that it can no longer ward off these invaders.

The immune system is made up of the thymus gland, white blood cells, bone marrow, the spleen, lymph nodes and ducts, and various protein and polypeptide chemical weapons like antibodies and interferon. The thymus makes killer white blood cells called T-cells, and tells them what to attack and when. Without these instructions, the T-cells may not recognize the body's enemies, or they may mistake the body's cells for enemies and attack their own lines.

Before puberty, the thymus gland is large and highly active. If you could keep it functioning at that level, you could live for hundreds of years. After puberty, however, the thymus shrivels up and its high level of activity falls off. A major factor in this decline is the greatly reduced rate of release of growth hormone as we get older. Growth hormone is produced by the pituitary gland in the brain, and it is required by the thymus gland to function properly.

The answer of the pharmaceutical industry was a patentable form of growth hormone given to the elderly by injection. Preliminary results were encouraging. In elderly men injected with the drug, body fat decreased by 14 percent, lean body mass expanded by 9 percent, and skin thickness increased by 7 percent. Lung and heart functioning also improved. Unfortunately, the therapy costs $14,000 a year and has potential side effects, ranging from enlargement of the face and extremities to hypertension, arthritis and heart failure. There is also a possible increased risk of cancer.[7]

Again, there are safer, more natural options. A number of cheap, natural supplements will stimulate the release of growth hormone by the body without side effects.

Predominant among these is growth hormone's natural precursor, the amino acid L-*arginine*. The functional activity of the thymus can be measured by the circulating level of a hormonal factor produced by the thymus called thymulin. L-arginine has been shown to bring suppressed thymulin levels back to normal.[8] In 1992, Italian researchers showed that thirty days of oral arginine supplementation significantly increased the circulating level of thymulin both in elderly people and in patients with cancer.[9] In wounded rats, L-arginine actually stimulates wound healing better than an injection of growth hormone.[10] It also decreases cholesterol levels and atherogenesis (degenerative changes in the arteries) in both animals and humans.[11] L-arginine aids in liver and ammonia detoxification, collagen production, and in reversing kidney and liver disorders. Like growth hormone itself, it counteracts the effects of decreased metabolism on body fat, causing muscle mass to go up and body fat to go down.[12]

The amino acid L-*ornithine* is another growth hormone releaser, while the amino acid L-*cysteine* helps increase thymus function. Unfortunately, the amino acids may all soon be off the over-the-counter market, based on the L-tryptophan incident discussed in Chapter Thirteen. In Canada, they have already been removed from the shelves.

Other growth hormone releasers include peak exercise, fasting, and certain prescription drugs.[13] Supplements that increase the size of the thymus gland and its functional capacity include *vitamin A, vitamin C,* and *vitamin E,* and the minerals *zinc* and *selenium.*[14]

Another supplement that research shows to be an excellent rejuvenator is *DHEA* (dehydroepiandrosterone). DHEA is a hormone produced naturally by the adrenal glands, and like progesterone, it is a precursor to other hormones. (See Chapter One.) Blood levels of DHEA peak at around age twenty-five and drop dramatically by age seventy, suggesting the need for supplements. Supplemental DHEA can replace the waning hormones of men as well as women. As with natural progesterone, side effects are avoided because the tissues turn the precursor into active hormones only as needed.

In laboratory animals, DHEA improves memory and prevents obesity, diabetes, atherosclerosis, and breast cancer. Oral intake of DHEA reawakens thymus gland function, increasing the number of lymphocytes. It also permits serum cholesterol and other blood fats better entry into liver cells for excretion, effectively and quickly lowering serum cholesterol and triglyceride levels. In mice, DHEA has been found to *triple* the lifespan; and in humans, it's been shown to reverse symptoms of senility, diabetes, autoimmune disorders including rheumatoid arthritis, and Parkinson's disease.[15]

In 1985, DHEA was taken off the market by the FDA, but it has now been approved for over-the-counter sale and is available in health food stores. It is all the rage in some circles for menopausal complaints, but Dr. Walker has found in her practice that it is generally less effective than natural progesterone, perhaps because it is farther up on the hormone chain and winds up getting converted to adrenalin rather than to progesterone in women under stress.

If you had no access to supplements at all, you could still profoundly affect the length and quality of your retirement years by limiting what and how much you eat. In those regions of the world where a high percentage of the population approaches the century mark, the diet is rich in plant foods, low in flesh foods, and so low in calories that we would consider it inadequate. Average intakes run around 1500 calories a day. Animals kept on low-calorie diets also outlive those who eat more. Rats live about one-third longer when limited to 60 to 70 percent of their normal caloric intakes. Tumor growth is reduced by at least 30 percent in these animals, and breast cancer is practically eliminated.[16] The less you eat, the more time your body has to process what goes into it and clean house before being hit with another meal.

Luigi Cornaro, a fifteenth-century centenarian, maintained that the secret to living not only a long time but in health to the end was a "regular" life—simple, free of stress, and involving extremely frugal eating habits. He limited his daily intake to 12 ounces of food and 14 ounces of drink. He wrote at the age of ninety-five:

> Though at this great age, I am hearty and content, eating with a good appetite, and sleeping soundly. Moreover, all my senses are as good as ever. . . . How different from the life of most old men, full of aches and pains, and forebodings, whilst mine is a life of real pleasure.[17]

Chapter Eighteen

Stress, Sex, and Meditation

Such harmony is in immortal souls;
But whilst this muddy vesture of decay
Doth grossly close it in, we cannot hear it.
—*The Merchant of Venice*

Life in the fast lane is a chief contributor to the adrenal exhaustion of modern midlife women. Stress causes our much-needed progesterone to break down into other substances. It can also cause PMS in premenopausal women by raising estrogen levels.

Supplements—herbs, homeopathics, and natural hormones—all help. In addition, we can change our approach to stress. If we can't change the hand life deals us, we can change how we play it. Meditation, yoga, relaxation techniques, and biofeedback are aids in relaxing into our bodies.

Meditation can also substitute for the natural loss of sexual interest that comes with age. In India, the first twenty years of life are considered to be for education and play. The second twenty years are for bearing and rearing children and for supporting children and parents. After forty, the parent (at least if he is a man) is supported by his children while he retires to the woods and meditates and searches for God. Sexual urge is considered a positive hindrance to this quest, since Enlightenment comes only when the "Kundalini" fire has been re-routed from the genitals up the spinal cord to the "Third Eye."

Committed meditators attest that a good meditation can be just as satisfying as a good man. In fact some of the most ecstatic sensual experiences ever described by women come from the Christian mystics, who knew no men in the flesh at all. (Not that mystics of other religious persuasions haven't reached equivalent ecstatic heights; but the Christian mystics, whose visions centered on a personal relationship with God in human form, used the explicit language of sex.)

Meditation can also be an outlet for energies that are dissipated in sex. To quote Muktananda, a Hindu yogi who has influenced millions of Americans:

> Who knows what there is in this body! There are ... so many different springs welling with nectar, so many clusters of nerve filaments, so many kinds of musical harmonies, so many different fragrances; there are rays from so many different suns, abodes of so many different deities. Though all this is inside him, man, tragically caught in his delusion, indulges himself in the arid world outside.... The inner world is far greater than the outer world.[1]

When you no longer have the energy for the sexual exploits of your youth, you can look forward to turning that ardor to philosophical and religious study and meditation. You'll probably find you can sit still and concentrate better after forty than you could when you were young, perhaps due to the waning of those same hormones that keep young people on the prowl. And interest naturally turns to the Beyond as we see it gaining on us.

So how do you meditate? There are many techniques, but they all begin with total relaxation. Rammurti Mishra, M.D., in his book *Fundamentals of Yoga*, describes a three-step process: fixation, suggestion, and sensation.[2] First you fix your awareness on a part of your body (e.g. your legs). Then you suggest that they are relaxing. Then you feel the sensation you just suggested to yourself. ("I relax my legs, my legs are relaxing, my legs are totally relaxed.") The last stage, sensation or realization, is important. You must pause from your suggestions and feel that the suggestion has been accepted and manifested by the subconscious.

Other meditation teachers suggest following the intake and outlet of the breath. As you breathe out fully and deeply, your thoughts are let go. As a thought comes in, it is noted but not dwelled on. The object is to drop away from thoughts, to give the "chattering mind" a rest.

After you are totally relaxed, you can start suggesting and "realizing" positive auto-suggestions: perfect health, peace, love, confidence, dignity, faith, etc. Although the technique sounds like self-hypnotism, Dr. Mishra says "de-hypnotism" is a better word. In Indian theory, peace, love, bliss, and the other absolute virtues are our true natures. We have simply hypnotized ourselves into the limited view that we are less than we are. Meditation is the way to break this hypnotic spell and realize our true potential. Dr. Mishra asserts that eventually we will be able to conquer all pains and diseases simply by the dedicated practice of this ancient technique. Even if you never see heaven and angels, it shouldn't take long before you can feel waves of love and joy washing over your agitated menopausal soul.

The Christian version of the cosmic virtues Raja Yogis suggest to themselves is found in Philippians 4:8:

> Whatsoever things are true, whatsoever things are honest, whatsoever things are just, whatsoever things are pure, whatsoever things are lovely, whatsoever things are of good report; if there be any virtue, and if there be any praise, think on these things.

Meditation can also be a useful skill in preparation for growing older. Despite everything science has to offer, our bodies will eventually fall apart. The trick is to be able to fly free from the mortal shell when it's no longer functional. To quote from another meditation classic, Stewart Edward White's *Across the Unknown:*

> Fundamentally, life and all its experiences pass through you like radio waves, and you are not affected by them. It is only your resistance to them that damages you. Therefore if you can just let them pass through you, and assert yourself of higher

substance, you can take them in quantity, from the most exalted honors to the direst calamities. In themselves, they are as little disintegrating as shade on your body: they are just fleeting phenomena.[3]

Gerard Guillaume, M.D., a French physician who uses acupuncture to treat menopausal symptoms, observes:

A woman who has accepted her menopause attains inner peace, a serenity that prepares her to assume her own mortality. Resisted or rejected, menopause can initiate a chain of symptoms. Perhaps one can see here a basis for the frequent problems linked to menopause, especially in Occidental societies which reject the signs of aging. This dimension of menopause should lead us to consider that its treatment should not be reduced to a medical therapy only, whatever it might be, and that through menopause there is the possibility for reflection on life.[4]

True as far as it goes; but meditation can bring more than reflection on life and resignation to our fate. It can be a quite physical form of pleasure, a tuning in to the subtle feelings of the body in its most relaxed state. For these pleasurable feelings, however, you need to be healthy. Dr. Mishra says you can elevate your hormone levels just by meditating, but he also stresses that you can't meditate if you're not healthy. If hormone levels are elevated with supplements, both meditation and sexual enjoyment can be improved.

Dr. Peat suggests that pleasure itself has a hormonal component. He cites these cases:

A woman said, soon after she began using progesterone and thyroid, that, for the first time in her life she felt that her heart and abdomen were opening with feelings of love. Another said 'thyroid is love.' Since these women were using the hormones for problems that had developed gradually, over several years if not their entire life, the sudden change was dramatic. They had forgotten that life itself was pleasurable.

He adds, "Women who have had orgasms while taking thyroid have lost their sexual responsiveness when they stopped.... By improving life conditions (in many ways) the hormones of pleasure can have a bigger role in our physiology."[5]

Dr. Walker has seen hundreds of women whose lives have been transformed when natural remedies resolved their hormone imbalances. Women have sent her flowers to express their gratitude, a reward she never experienced while dispensing drugs at a hospital pharmacy.

In my own experience, both meditation and sex are heightened by appropriate doses of natural supplements, including progesterone, Chinese herbs, L-arginine, coenzyme Q10, vitamin E, Utrophin, or whatever seems warranted at the time. While Dr. Lee says natural progesterone may take weeks to build up sufficiently in the blood to eliminate hot flashes, it can positively affect sexual response in less than forty-eight hours. L-arginine is another supplement that can have a nearly immediate effect on sexual response (in larger doses, perhaps a teaspoon of the powdered form). Whether peak-oriented as in sex or expansive as in meditation, the pleasure response can be augmented by natural herbal, nutritional, and hormonal remedies.

Without the crisis of menopause, we might have missed those satisfying discoveries. The hormone changes of midlife can be the impetus for a newfound health, propelling us to find new, body-supporting solutions to vague discomforts we could ignore when they impinged less forcefully on our awareness. Menopause, like puberty, is a major life challenge for women. When met, it promises the reward of stable hormones and a body in balance. Combined with greater physical, emotional, and spiritual awareness, a sensitive understanding and support of our bodies' midlife changes can make the second half of our lives rich and rewarding.

Appendix

Products and Information: Where to Get Them

Alphabetical Listing of Outlets and Resources

ANNANDALE APOTHECARY
3299 Woodburn Rd.
Annandale, VA 22003
(703) 698-7411
[Homeopathic remedies, nutritional products, books]

APEX ENERGETICS
1701 E. Edinger Ave.
Santa Ana, CA 92705
(714) 973-7733
(714) 973-2238 FAX
[Homeopathic remedies for practitioners]

BELLE HAVEN PHARMACY, INC.
1451 Belle Haven Rd.
Alexandria, VA 22307
(703) 765-5656
(703) 765-6225 FAX
[Homeopathic remedies, kits,books; UPS delivery]

BHI (BIOLOGICAL HOMEOPATHIC INDUSTRIES)
11600 Cochiti S.E.
Albuquerque, NM 87123
(800) 621-7644
(505) 275-1672 FAX
[Combination homeopathic remedies]

BIOFORCE OF AMERICA LTD.
P.O. Box 507
Kinderhook, NY 12106
(800) 645-9135

BOERICKE & TAFEL (EAST COAST)
42 S. 15th St.
Philadelphia, PA 19102
(215) 569-4002
(215) 569-4255 FAX
[Homeopathic remedies, kits, books]

BOERICKE & TAFEL (WEST COAST)
2381 Circadian Way
Santa Rosa, CA 95407
(707) 571-8232
(707) 571-8237 FAX
[Homeopathic remedies, kits, books]

BOIRON USA (EAST COAST)
6 Campus Blvd., Bldg. A
Newton Square, PA 19073
(800) BOIRON-1 (264-7661)
(215) 532-8244 FAX
[Homeopathic remedies, kits, books, educational materials]

BOIRON USA (WEST COAST)
98C W. Cochran Street
Simi Valley, CA 93065
(800) BOIRON-1 (264-7661)
(805) 582-9091
(805) 582-9094 FAX
[Homeopathic remedies, kits, books]

BOTANICAL LABORATORIES
P.O. Box 1596
Ferndale, WA 98248
[NATRA-BIO/CLINICA herbal products]

BUDGET PHARMACY
3001 N.W. 7th St.
Miami, FL 33125
(800) 221-9772
[Homeopathic remedies, books, tapes]

DOLISOS AMERICA HOMEOPATHIC CO.
3014 Rigel Ave
Las Vegas, NV 89102
(702) 871-7153
(702) 871-9670 FAX
(800) 365-4767
[Homeopathic remedies]

ECLECTIC INSTITUTE
14385 Southeast Lusted Rd.
Sandy, OR 97055
(800) 332-4372
[Herbal products]

ECOLOGICAL FORMULAS
1061-B Shary Circle
Concord, CA 94518
[Ecological, Cardiovascular research products]

HANSON HOMEOPATHIC HERBAL MEDICINE
4540 Southside Blvd. #5
Jacksonville, FL 32216-5458
[Homeopathic remedies]

HEALTH CONCERNS
8001 Capwell Drive
Oakland, CA 94621
(510) 639-0280
(510) 639-9140 FAX
[Herbal products; Chinese Traditional Formulas]

HOMEOPATHIC EDUCATIONAL SERVICES
2124 Kittredge Street #N
Berkeley, CA 94704
(800) 359-9051 Mail Order
(510) 649-0294
[Books, tapes, software]

HOMEOPATHIC INFORMATIONAL RESOURCES, LTD.
Oneida River Park Drive
Clay, NY 13041
(800) 289-4447
[Books, homeopathic remedies, videos]

HYLANDS HOMEOPATHIC REMEDIES
See STANDARD HOMEOPATHIC COMPANY

JADE
East Earth Herb Inc.
P.O. Box 2802
Eugene, OR 97402
[Chinese herbal products and information]

K'AN HERBS
2425 Porter St. #18
Soquel, CA 95073
[Chinese herbal products]

LONGEVITY
9595 Wilshire Blvd. #502
Beverly Hills, CA 90212
[Homeopathic products]

LUYTIES PHARMACAL COMPANY/NU AGE LABORATORIES/FORMUR PUBLISHERS
4200 Laclede Ave.
St. Louis, MO 63108
(800) 325-8080
[Homeopathic remedies, kits, books]

MCZAND HERBAL
P.O. Box 5312
Santa Monica, CA 90409
(310) 822-0500
[Herbal products]

MADISON PHARMACY ASSOCIATES
429 Gammon Pl.
Madison, WI 53719
(800) 558-7046
[Oral micronized progesterone, vitamin and mineral supplements, books]

THE MEDICINE SHOPPE
6307 York Rd.
Baltimore, MD 21212-2699
(410) 323-1515
[Homeopathic remedies]

MERZ APOTHECARY, INC.
4716 N. Lincoln Ave.
Chicago, IL 60625
(800) 252-0275
(312) 989-0900
[Homeopathic and herbal remedies, books]

METAGENICS
971 Calle Negocio
San Clemente, CA 92673
[Herbal and vitamin products; ETHICAL NUTRIENTS products]

MID-AMERICA HOMEOPATHIC MEDICINE SHOP
P.O. Box 1275
Berkley, MI 48072
(800) 552-4956
[Homeopathic pharmacy]

NATIONAL CENTER FOR HOMEOPATHY
801 N. Fairfax St. #306
Alexandria, VA 22314
(703) 548-7790
(703) 548- 7792 (fax)
[Educational material; lists of practitioners in your area]

NATIONAL COLLEGE OF NATUROPATHIC MEDICINE
11231 S.E. Market Street
Portland, OR 97216
(503) 255-7355
[A national center for homeopathic education]

NATURE'S SECRET
For Health, Inc.
Denver General Mail Facility, Dept. 0704
Denver, CO 80263-0704
(800) 29 SECRET
[Ultimate Green, Ultimate Oil; herbs and vitamin products;
consumer information]

NATURE'S WAY PRODUCTS INC.
10 Mountain Spring Parkway
Springville, UT 84663
(801) 489-1500
[Herbal products]

NEW ENGLAND SCHOOL OF HOMEOPATHY
356 Middle Street
Amherst MA 01002
(203) 763-1225
[Courses, seminars, journals]

NEWTON LABORATORIES, INC.
612 Upland Trail
Conyers, GA 30207
(800) 448-7256
(404) 922-2644
[Homeopathic remedies, educational materials]

NF FORMULAS, INC.
805 S.E. Sherman
Portland, OR 97214
[Herbal, homeopathic and nutritional products]

OPTIMOX CORPORATION
P.O. Box 3378
Torrance, CA 90510-3378
(310) 618-9370
[OPTIVITE, GYNOVITE vitamin products]

PACIFIC RESEARCH LABORATORIES
1010 Crenshaw Blvd., Suite 170
Torrance, CA 90275
(310) 320-1132
(310) 320-7557 FAX
[Nutritional supplements, Yam Cream]

PHARMA BOTANIXX
9250 Jeronimo Road
Irvine, CA 92718
(800) 769-4372
[Chinese herbal formulas for women]

POWELL PHARMACY, INC.
11085 Little Patuxent Parkway
Columbia, MD 21044
(410) 997-1600
(301) 596-4071
[Homeopathic remedies, vitamins, referrals]

PROFESSIONAL HEALTH PRODUCTS
Nutritional Specialties Inc.
P.O. Box 80085
Portland, OR 97280
[Homeopathic and nutritional supplements;
PROBIOLOGICS products]

SEVEN FORESTS
U.S. Distribution
I.T.M. 2017 S.E. Hawthorne
Portland, OR 97214
[Chinese herbal products]

STANDARD HOMEOPATHIC CO.
210 W. 131st Street
Box 61067
Los Angeles, CA 90061
(800) 624-9659
(213) 321-4284
[Homeopathic remedies; complete selection of titles; JAIN
Indian homeopathic books]

SUN VALLEY HERB COMPANY
331 1st Avenue North
Ketchum, ID 83340
(208) 726-4790
[Lynne Walker, owner; herbs, homeopathic, menopausal
products]

TRANSITIONS FOR HEALTH
621 S.W. Alder St., Suite 900
Portland, OR 97205
(800) 888-6814
(800) 944-0168 FAX
[Pro-Gest, Es-Gen yam and soybean extracts in transdermal
cream or oil]

WASHINGTON HOMEOPATHIC PRODUCTS
4914 Del Ray Ave.
Bethesda, MD 20814
(800) 336-1695 (orders)
(301) 656-1695 or (301) 656-1847 (FAX)
[Homeopathic remedies]

WELEDA PHARMACY, INC.
175 N. Route 9W
Congers, NY 10920
(914) 268-8572
(914) 268-8574 FAX
[Homeopathic and anthroposophic remedies; mail orders]

WOMEN'S INTERNATIONAL PHARMACY
5708 Monona Dr.
Madison, WI 53716
(800) 279-5708
[Oral micronized progesterone]

Notes

Introduction to the Revised Edition

1. R. Rubin, "Estrogen anxiety," *U.S. News & World Report* (April 4, 1994), page 60.
2. The increased risk was 41% for women on HRT vs. 32% for women on estrogen alone. G. Colditz, et al., "The use of estrogens and progestins and the risk of breast cancer in postmenopausal women," *New England Journal of Medicine* 332:1589–93 (June 15, 1995). In a study reported in JAMA two weeks after the Colditz study, by contrast, no association was found between combined estrogen and progestin therapy (HRT) and breast cancer; but the number of long-term users was small. The authors conceded that if breast cancer requires ten or more years to become manifest, their study could not predict such an effect. See J. Stanford, et al., "Combined estrogen and progestin hormone replacement therapy in relation to risk of breast cancer in middle-aged women," *JAMA* 274(2):137–42 (July 12, 1995).
3. See S. Roan, "Study urges use of 2nd hormone in estrogen therapy," *Los Angeles Times*, Home Edition Part A, page 1 (February 7, 1996). The effectiveness of natural progesterone comes as no surprise. The reason the synthetics were proven before the natural version seems to have been simply that they were patentable and therefore had research funding from drug companies.
4. Writing Group for the PEPI Trial, "Effects of estrogen or estrogen/progestin regimens on heart disease risk factors in postmenopausal women," *JAMA* 273(3):199–208 (January 18, 1995).
5. C. Russell, "Gaining ground as the world's no. 1 killer," *Washington Post* (March 27–April 2, 1995), page 8.
6. Quoted in *Time* (June 26, 1995), pages 47–53.
7. M. Abramowicz, "New drugs for osteoporosis," *Medical Letter* (January 1, 1996), page 1; E. Tanouye, "Delicate balance: Estrogen study shifts ground for women — and for drug firms," *Wall Street Journal* (June 15, 1995), pages A1 ff.
8. H. Verhaar, et al., "A comparison of the action of progestins and estrogen on the growth and differentiation of normal adult human osteoblast-like cells in vitro," *Bone* 15(3):307–11 (1994). See also N.

Breslau, "Calcium, estrogen, and progestin in the treatment of osteo-porosis," *Rheumatic Disease Clinics of North America* 20(3):691–716 (August 1994).

9. B. Leibovitz, "Hatch-Richardson passes: No time to celebrate," *Townsend Letter for Doctors* 137:1306 (December 1994); "Alternative medicine and the law," *Townsend Letter for Doctors* 144:16–19 (July 1995).

10. "Wyeth-Ayerst makes additional milestone payment to Columbia Laboratories for regulatory approval of Crinone in France," *Miami Health-wire* (January 24, 1996).

11. P. Fripp, "Estrogen and Alzheimer's," *Harvard Women's Health Watch* 1:6 (July 1, 1994). See E. Barrett-Connor, et al, "Estrogen replacement therapy and cognitive function in older women," *JAMA* 269:1637–41 (1993) (Rancho Bernardo community: no link between estrogen and cognitive function); A. Paganini-Hill, "The risks and benefits of estrogen replacement therapy: Leisure World," *International Journal of Fertility and Menopausal Studies* 40 (Suppl 1):54–62 (1995) (estrogen users had reduced Alzheimer's risk); D. Brenner, et al., "Postmenopausal estrogen replacement therapy and the risk of Alzheimer's disease: A population-based case-control study," *American Journal of Epidemiology* 140(3):262–67 (1994) (no relation between estrogen use and risk of Alzheimer's).

12. P. Fripp, *op. cit.*

13. "Pap test standardization causing unnecessary biopsies," *HealthFacts* (March 1994), page 1.

14. See J. Fortner, "Inadvertent spread of cancer at surgery," *Journal of Surgical Oncology* 53:191–96 (1993); L. Harter, "Malignant seeding of the needle track during sterotaxic core needle breast biopsy," *Radiology* 185:713–14 (1992); F. Roussel, et al., "Evaluation of large-needle biopsy for the diagnosis of cancer," *Acta Cytologica* 39:449–52 (1995); F. Roussel, et al., "The risk of tumoral seeding in needle biopsies," *Acta Cytologica* 33(6):936–39 (1989); K. Denton, et al., "Secondary tumour deposits in needle biopsy tracks: An underestimated risk?", *Journal of Clinical Pathology* 43:82–84 (1990) ("[O]ne cannot automatically assume that there is no risk from fine needle aspiration or that such risks should be neglected. There are numerous examples, such as the one reported here of metastases to large needle tracks from renal and prostatic carcinomas, or from fine needle aspiration of pancreatic, lung, and pleural primaries. Clearly the risk, though small, is real...").

15. B. Rimer, "Putting the 'informed' in informed consent about mammography," *Journal of the National Cancer Institute* 87(10):703–04 (May 17, 1995).
16. A. Miller, "May we agree to disagree, or how do we develop guidelines for breast screening in women?", *Journal of the National Cancer Institute* 86(22):1729–31 (November 16, 1994) (emphasis added).
17. Dr. Gofman's report "Preventing Breast Cancer" is available from the Committee for Nuclear Responsibility, P.O. Box 421993, San Francisco, California 94142.
18. See M. Castleman, "Why?", *Mother Jones* (May 1, 1994), pages 34 ff.
19. M. Key, "Data on estrogens in soybeans may make ERT more acceptable," *Cancer Biotechnology Weekly* (October 23, 2995), page 10; E. Braverman, et al., "Natural estrogen and progesterone: Research indicates health benefits of natural vs. synthetic hormones," *Total Health* (October 1991), page 55.
20. C. Herman, et al., "Soybean phytoestrogen intake and cancer risk," *Journal of Nutrition* 125(3 Suppl):757S-770S (1995). See also A. Molteni, et al., "In vitro hormonal effects of soybean isoflavones," *Journal of Nutrition* 125 (3 Suppl):751S-756S (1995).
21. A. Boress, "Scientists spotlight phytoestrogens for better health," *Tufts University Diet & Nutrition Letter* 12:3 (February 1, 1995).
22. S. Pratt, "Body and soy: New study indicates soy-rich diet can lower cholesterol," *Chicago Tribune* (August 22, 1995).
23. A. Mullins, "Premarin: A bitter pill to swallow," *Healthy & Natural Journal* (vol. 2, issue 1).
24. *Ibid.*; S. Pratt, *op. cit.*
25. N. Shaw, et al., "A vegetarian diet rich in soybean products compromises iron status in young students," *Journal of Nutrition* 125:212–19 (1995).

Introduction. Feminine Forever

1. R. Wilson, *Feminine Forever* (New York: Lippincott, 1966), p. 17.
2. A. Skolnick, "At third meeting, menopause experts make the most of insufficient data," *JAMA* 268(18):2483–85 (November 11, 1992); J. Froom, "Selections from current literature: Hormone therapy in postmenopausal women," *Family Practice* 8(3):288–92 (1991).
3. See Chapter 4.
4. L. Huppert, "Hormonal replacement therapy: Benefits, risks, doses," *Medical Clinics of North America* 71(1):23–39 (1987).

5. See "Progesterone: Inelegant ingredient," *Menopause News* 2(6):1 (November/December 1992); G. Sheehy, *The Silent Passage: Menopause* (New York: Random House, 1991, 1992), p. 21.

6. See Chapter 4.

7. L. Nachtigall, M.D., et al., *Estrogen* (New York: Harper Collins, 1991), pp. 41, 169 (italics omitted).

8. "Drug R & D costs doubled in decade," *American Medical News* (May 18, 1990), pp. 3, 53. Counting the development costs of drugs that fail, the figure is substantially higher.

9. See, e.g., M. Mintz, "Lilly officials knew of deaths before U.S. approved drugs," *Washington Post* (July 22, 1983), p. A8; D. Foster, et al., "The illusion of safety Part One: Poisoned research," *Mother Jones* 7(5):38–49 (1982); "Implants in jaw joint fail, leaving patients in pain and disfigured," *Wall Street Journal* (August 31, 1993), pp. A1, A4.

10. P. Hilts, "Dangers of some new drugs go undetected, study says," *New York Times* (May 27, 1990).

11. J. Calfee, "The FDA vs. the First Amendment," *Townsend Letter for Doctors* (August/September 1992), pp. 679–80 (reprinted from the *New York Times*).

12. See Chapter 9.

13. D. Eisenberg, et al., "Unconventional medicine in the United States," *New England Journal of Medicine* 328:246–52 (1993).

Chapter One. Was It Really Supposed to Be This Way?

1. D. Shefrin, N.D., T. Hudson, N.D., "Menopause," audiotape (Naturopathic Educational Series, tele. 800–743–2256); "Phytotherapy review & commentary," *Townsend Letter for Doctors* (May 1992), p. 434.

2. H. Aldercreutz, et al., "Dietary estrogens and the menopause in Japan," *Lancet* 339:1233 (1992).

3. Y. Beyenne, "Cultural significance and physiological manifestations of menopause: A biocultural analysis," *Culture, Med. Psychiatry* 10:58 (1986).

4. See Chapter 14.

5. H. Aldercreutz, et al., *op. cit.*

6. L. Swartzman, et al., "Impact of stress on objectively recorded menopausal hot flushes and on flush report bias," *Health Psychology* 9(5): 529–45 (1990).

Chapter Two. A Question of Balance

1. See K. Keville, "A total approach to fighting PMS," *Vegetarian Times* (August 1986), pp. 40 ff.
2. D. Williams, "The forgotten hormone," *Alternatives for the Health Conscious Individual* 4(6):41–46 (December 1991).
3. *Ibid.*
4. R. Peat, *Nutrition for Women* (Eugene, Oregon: Kenogen, 1981), p. 40.
5. *Ibid.*, pp. 11 and 22, citing sources including A. Lipschutz, *Steroid Hormones and Tumors* (Baltimore: Williams and Wilkens Co., 1950).
6. *Ibid.*, p. 3.
7. G. Griffin, *World Without Cancer* (Westlake Village, California: American Media, 1974), pp. 79–82.
8. R. Peat, *op. cit.*, p. 3.
9. See note 5.
10. R. Peat, *op. cit.*, pp. 11–21; J. Lee, M.D., "Significance of molecular configuration specificity: The case of progesterone and osteoporosis," *Townsend Letter for Doctors* 119:558–62 (1993).
11. J. Prior, "Progesterone as a bone-trophic hormone," *Endocrine Reviews* 11(2):386–98 (1990).
12. R. Peat, *op. cit.*, pp. 6 and 17–18.
13. J. Lee, M.D., "Slowing the aging process with natural progesterone" (Sebastopol, California; unpublished research paper).
14. R. Peat, "Progesterone in orthomolecular medicine," unpublished research paper (available from Foundation for Hormonal and Nutrition Research, 8150 S.W. Barnes Rd., Portland, Oregon 97225), pp. 30–31, citing O. Warburg, *The Metabolism of Tumors* (New York: R.R. Smith, Inc., 1931), M. Gerson, *A Cancer Therapy* (New York: Whittier Books, 1958), and I. Tallberg, *Protides of the Body Fluids* (1978).
15. D. Rubinow, et al., "Changes in plasma hormones across the menstrual cycle in patients with mentally related mood disorder and in control subjects," *American Journal of Obstetrics and Gynecology* 158(1):5–11 (1988).

Chapter Three. Menopause and the Drug Revolution

1. "Making medicine, making money," *Philadelphia Inquirer* (December 1992), quoted in "If they only knew ...," *Homeopathy Today* (March 1993), p. 23.
2. P. Stumpf, "Pharmacokinetics of estrogen," *Obstetrics and Gynecology* 75:9S–14S (1990).

3. R. Peat, "Origins of progesterone therapy," *Townsend Letter for Doctors* (November 1992), pp. 1016–17; R. Sitruk-Ware, et al., "Oral micronized progesterone," *Contraception* 36(4):373–402 (1987).

4. J. Healey, "The cancer weapon America needs most," *Reader's Digest* (June 1992), pp. 69–72.

5. L. Huppert, "Hormonal replacement therapy: Benefits, risks, doses," *Medical Clinics of North America* 71(1):23–39 (1987).

6. M. Whitehead, et al., "The role and use of progestogens," *Obstetrics and Gynecology* 75(4):59S–76S (1990).

7. R. Sitruk-Ware, et al., *op. cit.*

8. G. Sheehy, *The Silent Passage: Menopause* (New York: Random House, 1991, 1992), pp. 18–19.

9. *Ibid.*; S. Whitcroft, et al., "Hormone replacement therapy: Risks and benefits," *Clinical Endocrinology* 36:15–20 (1992); N. Lauersen, M.D., *PMS: Premenstrual Syndrome and You* (New York: Simon & Schuster, 1983).

10. M. Whitehead, *op. cit.*

11. A. Skolnick, "At third meeting, menopause experts make the most of insufficient data," *JAMA* 268(18):2483–85 (November 11, 1992).

12. L. Nachtigall, M.D., et al., *Estrogen* (New York: Harper Collins Publishers, 1991), p. 169.

Chapter 4. Cancer, Heart Disease and Osteoporosis: Are We Trading One Disease for Another?

1. A. Skolnick, "At third meeting, menopause experts make the most of insufficient data," *JAMA* 268(18):2483–85 (November 11, 1992).

2. R. Peat, *Nutrition for Women* (Eugene, Oregon: Kenogen, 1981), p. 45.

3. B. Henderson, et al., "Estrogen use and cardiovascular disease," *American Journal of Obstetrics and Gynecology* 154:1181–86 (1986).

4. M. Walker, "Breast cancer and the new post-mastectomy prosthesis," *Townsend Letter for Doctors* 119:566–69 (June 1993).

5. J. Froom, "Selections from current literature: Hormone therapy in postmenopausal women," *Family Practice* 8(3):288–92 (1991).

6. "Progesterone: Inelegant ingredient," *Menopause News* 2(6):1 (November/December 1992). See also G. Sheehy, *The Silent Passage: Menopause* (New York: Random House, 1991, 1992), p. 21.

7. J. Calfee, "The FDA vs. the First Amendment," *New York Times*, reprinted in *Townsend Letter for Doctors* 109/110:679–80 (August/September 1992).

8. *Ibid.*
9. A. Skolnick, *op. cit.*
10. See T. Bush, et al., "Cardiovascular mortality and noncontraceptive use of estrogen in women," *Circulation* 75(6):1102–09 (1987); M. Stampfer, et al., "A prospective study of postmenopausal estrogen therapy and coronary heart disease," *New England Journal of Medicine* 313:1044–49 (1985); K. Hunt, et al., "Mortality in a cohort of long-term users of hormone replacement therapy: An updated analysis," *British Journal of Obstetrics and Gynaecology* 97:1080–86 (1990); R. Ross, et al., "Menopausal estrogen therapy and protection from death from ischaemic heart disease," *Lancet* (April 18, 1981), pp. 858–60.
11. S. Cummings, "Evaluating the benefits and risks of postmenopausal hormone therapy," *American Journal of Medicine* 91(58):14S–19S (1991). See also W. Utian, quoted in A. Skolnick, *op. cit.*
12. K. Hunt, et al., *op. cit.*
13. M. Stampfer, et al., *op. cit.*
14. P. Wilson, et al., "Postmenopausal estrogen use, cigarette smoking, and cardiovascular morbidity in women over 50," *New England Journal of Medicine* 313:1038–43 (1985).
15. See J. Froom, *op. cit.*
16. See L. Huppert, "Hormonal replacement therapy: Benefits, risks, doses," *Medical Clinics of North America* 71(1):23–39 (1987).
17. R. Peat, "Estrogen in 1990," *Blake College Newsletter* (Eugene, Oregon).
18. R. Peat, *Nutrition for Women*, pp. 44 and 49, citing S. Shapiro, "Oral contraceptives: A time to take stock," *New England Journal of Medicine* 315:450 (1986); Seelig and Heggtveit, *American Journal of Clinical Nutrition* 27:59–79 (1974); and many other studies. See also S. Lark, M.D., *Menopause Self Help Book* (Berkeley, California: Celestial Arts, 1990, 1992), p. 221.
19. See U. Ottosson, et al., "Subfractions of high-density lipoprotein cholesterol during estrogen replacement therapy: A comparison between progestogens and natural progesterone," *Journal of Obstetrics and Gynecology* 151:746–50 (1985); G. Silferstolpe, et al., "Lipid metabolic studies in oophorectomised women: Effects of three different progestogens," *Acta Obstetrica et Gynecologica Scandinavica* [Suppl.] 88:89–95 (1979); E. Hirvonen, et al., "Effects of different progestogens on lipoproteins during postmenopausal replacement therapy," *New England Journal of Medicine* 304:560–63 (1981). For studies in which added progestogens

had no significant effect on lipoprotein levels, see C. Christiansen, et al., "Five years with continuous combined oestrogen/progestogen therapy," *British Journal of Obstetrics and Gynaecology* 97:1087–92 (1990); and K. Hunt, et al., *op. cit.*

20. *Physician's Desk Reference* (Oradell, New Jersey: Medical Economics Co., 1989), p. 2356.

21. "Transdermal estrogen," *Medical Letter* 28(728):119–20 (1986); "Patching up older bones," *Harvard Health Letter* 17(12):8 (October 1992); P. Stumpf, "Pharmacokinetics of estrogen," *Obstetrics and Gynecology* 75:9S–14S (1990); J. Sachs, *What Women Should Know About Menopause* (New York: Dell Publishing, 1991), p. 63.

22. J. Sullivan, et al., "Estrogen replacement and coronary artery disease," *Archives of Internal Medicine* 150:2557–62 (1990).

23. *Ibid.;* C. Danielson, et al., "Hip fractures and fluoridation in Utah's elderly population," *JAMA* 268(6):746–48 (August 12, 1992).

24. J. Reginster, et al., "Prevention of postmenopausal bone loss by tiludronate," *Lancet* (December 23/30, 1989), pp. 1469–71.

25. L. Huppert, *op. cit.*

26. U. Barzel, "Estrogens in the prevention and treatment of postmenopausal osteoporosis: A review," *American Journal of Medicine* 85:847–50 (1988).

27. M. Walker, *op. cit.*

28. L. Goodman, et al., *Pharmacological Basis of Therapeutics* (New York: MacMillan Publishing Co., 1975), p. 1429.

29. *Physicians' Desk Reference, op. cit.,* p. 2180.

30. L. Bergkvist, et al., "The risk of breast cancer after estrogen and estrogen-progestin replacement," *New England Journal of Medicine* 321(5):293–97 (1989).

31. J. Scott, "Hormones may increase cancer risk, study says," *Los Angeles Times* (August 2, 1989), pp. I:1,15.

32. G. Colditz, et al., "Type of postmenopausal hormone use and risk of breast cancer: 12-year follow-up from the Nurses' Health Study," *Cancer Causes and Control* 3:433–39 (1992).

33. R. Gambrell, et al., "Decreased incidence of breast cancer in postmenopausal estrogen-progestogen users," *Obstetrics and Gynecology* 62(4):435–43 (1983).

34. W. Dupont, et al., "Menopausal estrogen replacement therapy and breast cancer," *Archives of Internal Medicine* 151:67–72 (1991).

35. See discussion in G. Colditz, et al., "Prospective study of estrogen

replacement therapy and risk of breast cancer in postmenopausal women," *JAMA* 264(20):2648–53 (1990), at 2652. The three studies involving more than 100 cases were P. Mills, "Prospective study of exogenous hormone use and breast cancer in Seventh-day Adventists," *Cancer* 64:591–97 (1989) (current users of ERT had a 69% increase in breast cancer risk); K. Hunt, et al., "Long-term surveillance of mortality and cancer incidence in women receiving hormone replacement therapy," *British Journal of Ostetrics and Gynecology* 94:620–35 (1987); and a ten-year followup of the Nurses' Health Study showing a 36% greater risk for estrogen users.

36. G. Colditz, et al., *op. cit.* (1990 and 1992 articles).
37. M. Sillero-Arenas, et al., "Menopausal hormone replacement therapy and breast cancer: A meta-analysis," *Obstetrics and Gynecology* 79(2): 286–93 (1992).
38. C. Yang, et al., "Noncontraceptive hormone use and risk of breast cancer," *Cancer Causes and Control* 3(5):475–79 (1992).
39. L. Bergvist, et al., *op. cit.*
40. M. Stampfer, et al., *op. cit.*
41. L. Huppert, *op. cit.*
42. U. Barzel, *op. cit.*
43. A. Skolnick, *op. cit.*
44. L. Zussman, et al, "Sexual response after hysterectomy-oophorectomy: Recent studies and reconsideration of psychogenesis," *American Journal of Obstetrics and Gynecology* 140(7):725–29 (1981).

Chapter Five. Primary Prevention: Menopause by Surgery and Drugs

1. L. Dennerstein, et al., *Gynaecology, Sex and Psyche* (Melbourne: Melbourne University Press, 1978), p. 166.
2. V. Hufnagel, M.D., *No More Hysterectomies* (New York: Penguin Books, 1989), pp. 59–67.
3. G. Colditz, et al., "Menopause and the risk of coronary heart disease in women," *New England Journal of Medicine* 316(18):1105–10 (1987).
4. V. Hufnagel, *op. cit.*
5. *Ibid.*, citing *Arch. Gynaekol* 35:1 (1989).
6. E. Munnell, "Total hysterectomy," *American Journal of Obstetrics and Gynecology* 54:31 (1947).
7. L. Zussman, et al, "Sexual response after hysterectomy-oophorectomy: Recent studies and reconsideration of psychogenesis," *American Journal of Obstetrics and Gynecology* 140(7):725–29 (1981).

8. See, e.g., M. Kobayashi, et al., "Immunohistochemical localization of pituitary gonadotrophins and estrogen in human postmenopausal ovaries," *Acta Obstetrica et Gynecologica Scandinavica* 72:76–80 (1993).

9. V. Hufnagel, *op. cit.*; W. Utian, "Effect of hysterectomy, oophorectomy and estrogen therapy on libido," *International Journal of Gynaecology and Obstetrics* 13:97 (1975); "Dr. John Lee speaking on natural progesterone, 1992," audiotape (Sebastopol, California).

10. A. Kinsey, *Sexual Behavior in the Human Female* (Philadelphia: W.B. Saunders Co., 1953).

11. Quoted in L. Zussman, et al., *op. cit.*

12. V. Hufnagel, *op. cit.*, pp. 108, 117; S. Lark, M.D., *Menopause Self Help Book* (Berkeley, California: Celestial Arts, 1990, 1992), pp. 220–21.

13. See "Breast cancer—Have we lost our way?" [editorial], reprinted from *The Lancet* in *Townsend Letter for Doctors*, 118:477–78 (May 1993).

14. A. Fugh-Berman, "Tamoxifen on trial: The high risks of prevention," *The Nation* (December 21, 1992).

15. *Ibid.*

16. See R. Moss, *The Cancer Industry: Unravelling the Politics* (New York: Paragon House, 1989), p. 369 and generally.

17. *Ibid.*

Chapter Six. Early Detection: Prevention" That Can Spread the Disease

1. R. Moss, *The Cancer Industry: Unravelling the Politics* (New York: Paragon House, 1989), p. 16.

2. "Author of Canadian breast cancer study retracts warnings," *Journal of the National Cancer Institute* 84(11):832–34 (June 3, 1992).

3. A. Miller, et al., "Canadian National Breast Screening Study: 1. Breast cancer detection and death rates among women aged 40 to 49 years," *Canadian Medical Association Journal* 147(10):1459–76 (1992).

4. A. Miller, "Re: 'Author of Canadian breast cancer study retracts warnings'," *Journal of the National Cancer Institute* 84(17):1365–70 (1992).

5. P. Skrabanek, "False premises and false promises of breast cancer screening," *Lancet* (August 10, 1985), pp. 316–20.

6. R. Moss, *op. cit.*, pp. 32–33; M. Kushi, *The Cancer Prevention Diet* (New York: St. Martin's Press, 1983), p. 79.

7. H. Bloom, "The influence of delay on the natural history and prognosis of breast cancer," *British Journal of Cancer* 19:228–62 (1965).

8. "Breast cancer—Have we lost our way?", *Lancet,* reprinted in *Townsend Letter for Doctors* 118:477–79 (May 1993).
9. R. Moss, *op. cit.,* p. 33 (figures are age-adjusted and take into account that life expectancy has increased).
10. M. Walker, "Breast cancer and the new post-mastectomy prosthesis," *Townsend Letter for Doctors* 119:566–69 (June 1993).
11. "New cancer statistics show losses, gains," *Journal of the National Cancer Institute* 82(15):1238 (1990), quoting Brenda Edwards, Ph.D., acting associate director of NCI's Surveillance Program.
12. See G. Cowley, et al., "In pursuit of a terrible killer," *Newsweek* (December 10, 1990), pp. 66–68.
13. P. Skrabanek, *op. cit.*
14. Quoted in B. Lynes, *The Healing of Cancer* (Queensville, Ontario: Marcus Books, 1989), p. 151.
15. *Ibid.,* pp. 151–52.
17. E. Robin, M.D., *Matters of Life & Death: Risks vs. Benefits of Medical Care* (New York: W. H. Freeman and Co., 1984), pp. 130, 142–43.
17. T. Mygind, et al., "Mammography is an objective diagnostic method," *Acta Rad. [Diagn.]* 25:189–93 (1984).
18. J. Devitt, "False alarms of breast cancer," *Lancet* (November 25, 1989), pp. 1257–58.
19. *Ibid.*
20. A. Miller, et al., "Canadian National Breast Screening Study: 2. Breast cancer detection and death rates among women aged 50 to 59 years," *Canadian Medical Association Journal* 147(10):1477–88 (1992).
21. L. Barbach, Ph.D., *The Pause* (New York: Penguin Books, 1993), p. 135.
22. L. Nachtigall, M.D., et al., *Estrogen* (New York: Harper Collins Publishers, 1991), pp. 20, 184–85; J. Sachs, *What Women Should Know About Menopause* (New York: Dell Publishing, 1991), p. 59.
23. J. McCormick, "Cervical smears: A questionable practice?", *Lancet* (July 22, 1989), pp. 207–09.
24. M. Kelley, "Hypercholesterolemia: The cost of treatment in perspective," *Southern Medical Journal* 83:1421–25 (1990).
25. See E. Robin, *op. cit.*

Chapter Seven. Herbs East and West

1. Computer drawing by Lynne Walker and Jamie Brown.
2. B. Flaws, *My Sister the Moon: The Diagnosis and Treatment of Menstrual*

Diseases by Traditional Chinese Medicine (Boulder, Colorado: Johnson Books, 1992), pp. 314–15.

3. See, e.g., J. Shaw, "Aging process and anti-aging effects of Chinese herbal medicines," *International Journal of Chinese Medicine* 1:45–48 (1984); *Herbal Pharmacology in the People's Republic of China: A Trip Report of the American Pharmacology Delegation* (Washington D.C.: National Academy of Sciences, 1975); J. Chen, "'Pharmacology,' medicine and public health in the People's Republic of China," DHEW Publication No. (NIH) 72–67, pp. 93–108 (1972); Kiangsu New Medical College, *Pharmacopoeia of Chinese Drugs (Chung Yao Ta Zi Tien)* (Shanghai: People's Publishing House, 1977) (in Chinese).

4. J. Chen, "Pharmacologic actions and therapeutic uses of Ginseng and Tang Kwei," *International Journal of Chinese Medicine* 1(3):23–27 (1984).

5. *Ibid.*

6. D. Bensky, et al., *Chinese Herbal Medicine: Materia Medica* (Seattle: Eastland Press, 1986), p. 476.

7. E. Duker, et al., "Effects of extracts from *Cimicifuga racemosa* on gonadotropin release in menopausal women and ovariectomized rats," *Planta Medica* 57:420–24 (1991).

8. P. Holmes, *The Energetics of Western Herbs* (Boulder, Colorado: Artemis, 1989), pp. 471–73.

9. K. Keville, "A total approach to fighting PMS," *Vegetarian Times* (August 1986), pp. 40 ff.

10. See P. Holmes, *op. cit.*, pages 236, 707; G. Guillaume, "Postmenopausal osteoporosis and Chinese medicine," *American Journal of Acupuncture* 20(2):105–11 (1992).

11. J. Morgenthaler, et al., eds., *Stop the FDA* (Menlo Park, California: Health Freedom Publications, 1992), pp. 67, 73–74.

Chapter Eight. Homeopathic Remedies

1. W. Ludwig, "Fundamental principles of Mora Therapy" [reprint of lecture, undated].

2. See H. Coulter, *Divided Legacy: The Conflict Between Homeopathy and the American Medical Association*, Vol. III (Berkeley, California: North Atlantic Books, 1982, 2d ed.); M. Weiner, et al., The *Complete Book of Homeopathy* (Garden City Park, New York: Avery Publishing Group Inc., 1989); M. Kaufman, *Homeopathy in America: The Rise and Fall of a Medical Heresy* (Baltimore: Johns Hopkins Press, 1971); B. Inglis, *Natural Medicine* (Glasgow: William Collins Sons and Company Ltd., 1979).

3. In re *George A. Guess*, 393 S.E.2d 833 (1990).

4. F. Royal, "Homeopathy and EDT: Upheld by modern science—with case histories," *American Journal of Acupuncture* 20(1):55–65 (1992).

5. M. Beckerich, "Appetoff: Another diet fad," *Veterinary and Human Toxicology* 31(6):540–43 (1989).

6. M. Browne, "Controversial report in *Nature* supports homeopathy," *Townsend Letter for Doctors* (August/September 1988), p. 378; D. Ullman, "Recent homeopathic research startles scientists," *ibid.*, p. 335.

7. D. Ullman, *ibid.* See, e.g., P. Fisher, et al., "The effect of homeopathic treatment on fibrositis," *British Medical Journal* 299:365–66 (1989); J. Ferley, et al., "A controlled evaluation of a homeopathic preparation in the treatment of influenza-like symptoms," *British Journal of Clinical Pharmacology* 27:329–35 (1989); D. Reilly, et al., "Is homeopathy a placebo response?," *Lancet* (October 1986), pp. 881–86.

8. B. Borho, "Therapy of the menopausal syndrome with Mulimen—Results of a multicentre post-marketing survey," *Biological Therapy* 10(2):226–29 (1992).

9. Material summarized from W. Boericke, M.D., *Homeopathic Materia Medica* (Philadelphia: Boericke & Runyon, 1927), and R. Morrison, M.D., *Desktop Guide to Keynotes and Confirmatory Symptoms* (Albany, California: Hahnemann Clinic Publishing, 1993).

Chapter Nine. Rebuilding Your Bones

1. J. Lee, "Osteoporosis reversal: The role of progesterone," *International Clinical Nutrition Review* 10(3):384–91 (1990); J. Lee, "Significance of molecular configuration specificity: The case of progesterone and osteoporosis," *Townsend Letter for Doctors* 119:558–62 (1993).

2. R. Peat, "Origins of progesterone therapy," *Townsend Letter for Doctors* (November 1992), pp. 1016–17.

3. *Ibid.*; M. Whitehead, et al., "The role and use of progestogens," *Obstetrics and Gynecology* 75:59S–76S (1990).

4. R. Peat, *op. cit.*; J. Lee, M.D., "Slowing the aging process with natural progesterone" (Sebastopol, California; unpublished research paper); R. Peat, *Nutrition for Women* (Eugene, Oregon: Kenogen, 1981), p. 25; L. Huppert, "Hormonal replacement therapy: Benefits, risks, doses," *Medical Clinics of North America* 71(1):23–39 (1987).

5. J. Lee, "Osteoporosis reversal," *op. cit.*; J. Lee, "Is natural progesterone the missing link in osteoporosis prevention and treatment?", *Medical Hypotheses* 35:314–16 (1991).

6. J. Lee, "Osteoporosis reversal," *op. cit.*; J. Lee, "Significance of molecular configuration specificity," *op. cit.*

7. J. Lee, "Successful menopausal osteoporosis treatment: Restoring osteoclast/osteoblast equilibrium" (Sebastopol, California; unpublished research paper); "Dr. John Lee speaking on natural progesterone," audiotape (Sebastopol: BLL Publishing, 1992).

8. P. Rylance, et al., "Natural progesterone and antihypertensive action," *British Medical Journal* 290:13–14 (1985); E. Darj, et al., "Clinical and endometrial effects of oestradiol and progesterone in post-menopausal women," *Maturitas* 13:109–15 (1991).

9. G. Lane, et al., "Dose dependent effects of oral progesterone on the estrogenised postmenopausal endometrium," *British Medical Journal* 287:1241–45 (1983); E. Darj, et al., *op. cit.*

10. U. Ottosson, et al., "Subfractions of high-density lipoprotein cholesterol during estrogen replacement therapy: A comparison between progestogens and natural progesterone," *American Journal of Obstetrics and Gynecology* 151:746–50 (1985); J. Hargrove, et al., "Menopausal hormone replacement therapy with continuous daily oral micronized estradiol and progesterone," *Obstetrics and Gynecology* 73:606–12 (1989).

11. See J. Prior, "Progesterone as a bone-trophic hormone," *Endocrine Reviews* 11(2):386–98 (1990).

12. J. Lee, "Successful osteoporosis treatment," *op. cit.*. Dr. Lee states that before 1976, when estrogen was routinely used alone, the means for adequate measurement of bone density were not available.

13. Adapted from J. Lee, "Slowing the aging process with natural progesterone," *op. cit.*

14. J. Lee, *Medical Hypotheses*, *op. cit.*; J. Lee, "Osteoporosis reversal," *op. cit.*; J. Prior, *op. cit.*

15. R. Peat, *Nutrition for Women*, *op. cit.*, p. 18.

16. *Ibid.*, p. 43; Lita Lee, Ph.D., "Estrogen, progesterone and female problems," *Earthletter* 1(2):1–4 (June 1991).

17. *Nutrition for Women*, *op. cit.*, p. 44; J. Lee, *Townsend Letter for Doctors*, *op. cit.*J. Lee, audiotape, *op. cit.*; J. Lee, "Understanding osteoporosis" (Sebastopol, California; unpublished research paper).

18. "Understanding osteoporosis," *op. cit.*; R. Peat, "Progesterone: Essential to your well-being," *Let's Live* (April 1982).

19. *Nutrition for Women*, *op. cit.*, pp. 6, 17 and 40, citing Strickler, *Contemporary Ob/Gyn* (August 1976).

20. *Ibid.*, p. 40.

21. J. Lee, audiotape, *op. cit.*
22. W. Utian, "Effect of hysterectomy, oophorectomy and estrogen therapy on libido," *International Journal of Gynaecology and Obstetrics* 13:97 (1975).
23. *Nutrition for Women, op. cit.*, pp. 11–12.
24. J. Lee, "Slowing the aging process," *op. cit.*
25. N. Lauersen, M.D., *PMS: Premenstrual Syndrome and You* (New York: Simon & Schuster, 1983); D. Shefrin, N.D., "Premenstrual syndrome and progesterone therapy," audiotape (Naturopathic Educational Series, tele. 800–743–2256).
26. *Nutrition for Women, op. cit.*, p. 43, citing the *Journal of Steroid Biochemistry*; J. Lee, *Townsend Letter for Doctors, op. cit.*
27. J. Lee, *ibid.*; J. Lee, "Slowing the aging process," *op. cit.*
28. J. Lee, "Fighting osteoporosis with natural progesterone," *op. cit.*. See also *Natural Progesterone: The Multiple Roles of a Remarkable Hormone*, BLL Publishg, P.O. Box 2068, Sebastopol, CA 95473.

Chapter Ten. Progesterone Therapy from PMS to Menopause

1. The Endometriosis Association, Milwaukee, "Facts and figures on endometriosis," *U.S. Pharmacist*, p. 42 (February 1993).
2. L. Graham, "Do you have a hormone shortage?", *Redbook* (February 1989), p. 16.
3. V. Hufnagel, M.D., *No More Hysterectomies* (New York: Penguin Books 1989), p. 126.
4. L. Graham, *op. cit.*, citing infertility specialist Jerome H. Check, M.D., Associate Professor of Obstetrics and Gynecology at Thomas Jefferson University in Philadelphia.
5. "Dr. John Lee speaking on natural progesterone, 1992," audiotape (Sebastopol: BLL Publishing, 1992).
6. L. Dusky, "Progesterone: Safe antidote for PMS," *McCall's* (October 1990), pp. 152–56.
7. R. Peat, "Progesterone: Essential to your well-being," *Let's Live* (April 1982).
8. G. Robinson, et al., "Problems in the treatment of premenstrual syndrome," *Canadian Journal of Psychiatry* 35:199–206 (1990), citing studies.
9. *Ibid.* See also H. Chihal, "Indications for drug therapy in premenstrual syndrome patients," *Journal of Reproductive Medicine* 32(6):449–52 (1987); E. Freeman, et al., "Ineffectiveness of progesterone suppository treatment for premenstrual syndrome," *JAMA* 264(3):349–53 (1990).

10. R. Peat, "Effectiveness of progesterone assimilation for the relief of premenstrual syndrome" (Eugene, Oregon; unpublished research paper).

11. L. Dennerstein, et al., "Progesterone and the premenstrual syndrome: A double blind crossover trial," *British Medical Journal* 290:1617–21 (1985).

12. L. Dusky, *op. cit.*; D. Shefrin, N.D., "Premenstrual syndrome and progesterone therapy," audiotape (Naturopathic Educational Series, tele. 800–743–2256); N. Lauersen, M.D., *PMS: Premenstrual Syndrome and You* (New York: Simon & Schuster, 1983).

13. J. Hargrove, et al., "Menopausal hormone replacement therapy with continuous daily oral micronized estradiol and progesterone," *Obstetrics and Gynecology* 73:606–12 (1989).

14. E. Darj, et al., "Clinical and endometrial effects of oestradiol and progesterone in post-menopausal women," *Maturitas* 13:109–15 (1991); G. Lane, et al., "Dose dependent effects of oral progesterone on the estrogenised postmenopausal endometrium," *British Medical Journal* 287:1241–45 (1983).

15. R. Sitruk-Ware, et al., "Oral micronized progesterone," *Contraception* 36(4):373–402 (1987).

16. J. Lee, audiotape, *op. cit.*

17. R. Peat, "Origins of progesterone therapy," *Townsend Letter for Doctors* 112:1016 (November 1992).

18. J. Lee, M.D., "Slowing the aging process with natural progesterone" (Sebastopol, California; unpublished research paper).

19. R. Peat, *Nutrition for Women* (Eugene, Oregon: Kenogen, 1981), p. 22.

20. L. Nachtigall, M.D., et al., *Estrogen* (New York: Harper Collins Publishers, 1991), pp. 45–46.

21. *Ibid.*, p. 26.

22. K. Dalton, "Prenatal progesterone and educational attainments," *British Journal of Psychiatry* 129:438–42 (1976).

Chapter Eleven. When You Need Estrogen

1. See Chapters 2 and 9.

2. V. Hufnagel, M.D., *No More Hysterectomies* (New York: Penguin Books, 1989), p. 38 (italics omitted).

3. Lita Lee, "Estrogen, progesterone and female problems," *Earthletter* 1(2):1–4 (June 1991).

4. See J. McDougall, M.D., "Balancing the estrogen issue," *Vegetarian Times* (August 1986), p. 44.

5. See Chapters 4 and 9.
6. V. Hufnagel, *op. cit.*, p. 138.
7. N. Lauersen, M.D., *PMS: Premenstrual Syndrome and You* (New York: Simon & Schuster 1983); Lita Lee, *op. cit.*; "Dr. John Lee speaking on natural progesterone, 1992," audiotape (Sebastopol, California); R. Peat, *Nutrition for Women* (Eugene, Oregon: Kenogen, 1981), pp. 11, 21.
8. D. Shefrin, N.D., T. Hudson, N.D., "Menopause," audiotape (Naturopathic Educational Series, tele. 800–743–2256).
9. See S. Lark, M.D., *Menopause Self Help Book* (Berkeley, California: Celestial Arts, 1990, 1992), p. 216.
10. A. Follingstad, "Estriol, the forgotten estrogen?", JAMA 239(1):29–30 (1978).
11. See L. Bergkvist, et al., "The risk of breast cancer after estrogen and estrogen-progestin replacement," *New England Journal of Medicine* 321(5):293–97 (1989).
12. "Transdermal estrogen," *Medical Letter* 28(728):119–20 (1986); "Patching up older bones," *Harvard Health Letter* 17(12):8 (October 1992); P. Stumpf, "Pharmacokinetics of estrogen," *Obstetrics and Gynecology* 75:9S–14S (1990).
13. Lita Lee, *op. cit.*
14. M. Beard, "Atrophic vaginitis: Can it be prevented as well as treated?" *Postgraduate Medicine* 91(6):257–60 (1992).
15. *Ibid.*; D. Shefrin, et al., *op. cit.*
16. M. Privette, et al., "Prevention of recurrent urinary tract infections in postmenopausal women," *Nephron* 50:24–27 (1988). See also J. Baldassarre, et al., "Special problems of urinary tract infection in the elderly," *Medical Clinics of North America* 75(2):375–90 (1991).
17. M. Privette, *ibid.*
18. I. Milsom, et al., "Vaginal immunoglobulin A (IgA) levels in postmenopausal women: Influence of oestriol therapy," *Maturitas* 13(2):129–35 (1991).
19. B. Eriksen, et al., "Urogenital estrogen deficiency syndrome: Investigation and treatment with special reference to hormone substitution," *Tidsskrift for den Norske Laegeforening* 111(24):2949–51 (1991). See also U. Molander, et al., "Effect of oral oestriol on vaginal flora and cytology and urogenital symptoms in the post-menopause," *Maturitas* 12(2):113–20 (1990); D. Gerbaldo, et al., "Endometrial morphology after 12 months of vaginal oestriol therapy in post-menopausal women," *Maturitas* 13(4):269–74 (1991).

20. D. Shefrin, et al., *op. cit.*
21. L. Huppert, "Hormonal replacement therapy: Benefits, risks, doses," *Medical Clinics of North America* 71(1):23–39 (1987); D. Shefrin, et al., *op. cit.*

Chapter Twelve. Preserving Your Female Organs: Alternatives to Surgery

1. S. Lark, M.D., *Menopause Self Help Book* (Berkeley, California: Celestial Arts, 1990, 1992), pp. 220–21; V. Hufnagel, M.D., *No More Hysterectomies* (New York: Penguin Books, 1989), pp. 108, 117; J. Lee, M.D., "Slowing the aging process with natural progesterone" (Sebastopol: BLL Publishing, 1992).
2. V. Hufnagel, *op. cit.*, p. 108; L. Nachtigall, M.D., et al., *Estrogen* (New York: Harper Collins Publishers, 1991), p. 192.
3. V. Hufnagel, *op. cit.*, p. 124.
4. S. Tsao, et al., "Toxicities of trichosanthin and alpha-momorcharin, abortifacient proteins from Chinese medicinal plants, on cultured tumor cell lines," *Toxicon* 28(10):1183–92 (1990).
5. V. Hufnagel, *op. cit.*, p. 108.
6. J. Lee, *op. cit.*
7. Ibid.
8. V. Hufnagel, *op. cit.*, pp. 4–5, 59–64, 114.
9. R. Peat, *Nutrition for Women* (Eugene, Oregon: Kenogen, 1981), p. 17.
10. John Lee, M.D., personal letter to author, May 10, 1993.
11. J. Lee, "Osteoporosis reversal: The role of progesterone," *International Clinical Nutrition Review* 10(3): 384–91 (1990). Compare J. Franklyn, et al., "Long-term thyroxine treatment and bone mineral density," *Lancet* 340:9–13 (1992), finding no significant difference in bone mineral density between patients on thyroid treatment and controls. Thyroid supplementation itself is not detrimental. It is excess thyroid that does harm.
12. R. Peat, *op. cit.*, pp. 16–21.

Chapter Thirteen. Natural Mood Elevators

1. L. Dusky, "Progesterone: Safe antidote for PMS," *McCall's* (October 1990), pp. 152–56.
2. R. Peat, *Nutrition for Women* (Eugene, Oregon: Kenogen, 1981), pp. 7–8.
3. L. Barbach, Ph.D., *The Pause* (New York: Penguin Books, 1993), p. 37.

4. R. Peat, *op. cit.*, p. 21.
5. V. Hufnagel, M.D., *No More Hysterectomies* (New York: Penguin Books 1989), pp. 39–40, citing L. Dennerstein, et al., "Headache and sex hormone therapy," *Headache* 18:146 (1978); L. Zussman, et al., "Sexual response after hysterectomy-oophorectomy: Recent studies and reconsideration of psychogenesis," *American Journal of Obstetrics and Gynecology* (August 1981), p. 140.
6. D. Manders, "The curious continuing ban of L-tryptophan: The serotonin connection," *Townsend Letter for Doctors* (October 1992), pp. 880–81; Citizens for Health, "Prepare for the worst: FDA propaganda ready to barrage media," *ibid.* (August/September 1993), pp. 860–61.
7. G. Null, "Prozac, Eli Lilly and the FDA," *Townsend Letter for Doctors* (March 1993), pp. 1 ff.; "A Prozac backlash," *Newsweek* (April 1, 1991), pp. 64–67.
8. D. Manders, *op. cit.*; G. Null, *op. cit.*; Citizens for Health, *op. cit.*
9. M. Shangold, "Exercise in the menopausal woman," *Obstetrics and Gynecology* 75:53S–58S (1990).
10. R. Peat, *op. cit.*, p. 92.
11. "PMS? Let 'em eat carbs," *Vegetarian Times* (March 1990), p. 17.

Chapter Fourteen. Diet, Exercise, and Hormone Balance

1. See J. Stamler, "Population studies," in R. Levy, et al., eds., *Nutrition, Lipids, and Coronary Heart Disease* (New York: Raven Press, 1979), vol. 1, pp. 25–88; J. Berg, "Can nutrition explain the pattern of international epidemiology of hormone-dependent cancers?", *Cancer Research* 35:3345–50 (1975); P. Nair, "Diet, nutrition intake, and metabolism in populations at high and low risk for colon cancer," *American Journal of Clinical Nutrition* 40:880–86 (1984); T. Hirayama, "Epidemiology of breast cancer with special reference to the role of diet," *Preventive Medicine* 7:173–95 (1978); B. MacMahon, et al., "Oestrogen profiles of Asian and North American women," *Lancet* 2:900–02 (1971); H. Aldercreutz, et al., "Dietary estrogens and the menopause in Japan," *Lancet* 339:1233 (1992).
2. J. McDougall, M.D., "Balancing the estrogen issue," *Vegetarian Times* (August 1986), p. 44.
3. D. Williams, "The forgotten hormone," *Alternatives for the Health Conscious Individual* 4(6):41–46 (1991); "Dr. John Lee speaking on natural progesterone, 1992," audiotape (Sebastopol, California).
4. B. Goldin, et al., *op. cit.*

5. J. Schneider, et al., "Effects of obesity on estradiol metabolism: Decreased formation of nonuterotropic metabolites," *Obstetrical and Gynecological Survey* 38(10):616 (1980).

6. E. Brown, *With the Grain: Eat More, Weigh Less, Live Longer* (New York: Carroll & Graf, 1990).

7. B. Goldin, et al., "Estrogen excretion patterns and plasma levels in vegetarian and omnivorous women," *New England Journal of Medicine* 307:1542–47 (1982).

8. See "Less fat, more grain can ease breast pain," *Vegetarian Times* (May 1989), p. 11; "PMS? Let 'em eat carbs," *ibid.* (March 1990), p. 17.

9. L. Barbach, Ph.D., *The Pause* (New York: Penguin Books, 1993), p. 174, citing S. Weed, *Menopausal Years*.

10. H. Aldercreutz, et al., *op. cit.*

11. G. Wilcox, et al., "Oestrogenic effects of plant foods in postmenopausal women," *British Medical Journal* 301(6757):905–06 (1990).

12. H. Aldercreutz, et al., *op. cit.*

13. B. Goldin, et al., "Effect of diet on excretion of estrogens in pre- and postmenopausal women," *Cancer Research* 41:3771–73 (1981); L. Cohen, "Diet and cancer," *Scientific American* 257(5):42–48 (1987).

14. See Chapter 5.

15. L. Cohen, et al., *op. cit.*

16. T. Shultz, et al., "Nutrient intake and hormonal status of premenopausal vegetarian Seventh-Day Adventists and premenopausal nonvegetarians," *Nutrition and Cancer* 4(4):247–59 (1983); B. Howie, et al., "Dietary and hormonal interrelationships among vegetarian Seventh-Day Adventists and non-vegetarian men," *American Journal of Clinical Nutrition* 42:127–34 (1985); K. Carroll, "Experimental evidence of dietary factors and hormone-dependent cancers," *Cancer Research* 35:3374–83 (1975); P. Hill, et al., "Diet and endocrine-related cancer," *Cancer* 39:1820–26 (1977).

17. J. Berg, *op. cit.*

18. See, e.g., B. Goldin, et al., *op. cit.*; M. Rosenthal, et al., "Effects of a high-complex-carbohydrate, low-fat, low-cholesterol diet on levels of serum lipids and estradiol," *American Journal of Medicine* 78:23–27 (1985); P. Hill, et al., "Diet and urinary steroids in black and white North American men and black South African men," *Cancer Research* 39:5101–05 (1979); P. Hill, et al., "Gonadotrophin release and meat consumption in vegetarian women," *American Journal of Clinical Nutrition* 43:37–41 (1986).

19. B. Howie, et al., *op. cit.*; T. Shultz, et al., *op. cit.*

20. "Breast cancer and PCB's: A possible link," *Business Week* (April 6, 1992), p. 36.

21. S. Gaskill, et al., "Breast cancer mortality and diet in the United States," *Cancer Research* 39:3628–37 (1979); P. Stocks, "Breast cancer anomalies," *British Journal of Cancer* 24:633–43 (1970).

22. S. Gaskill, et al., *op. cit.*; T. Hirayama, *op. cit.*

23. See, e.g., Y. Cha-Chung, et al., "Arrest of mammary tumor growth in vivo by L-arginine," *Biochemical and Biophysical Research Communications* 95(3):1306–13 (1980); J. Weisburger, et al., "Prevention by arginine glutamate of the carcinogenicity of acetamide in rats," *Toxicology and Applied Pharmacology* 14:163–75 (1969); A. Barbul, "Arginine: Biochemistry, physiology, and therapeutic implications," *Journal of Parenteral and Enteral Nutrition* 10(2): 227–38 (1986).

24. S. Cummings, et al., "Epidemiology of osteoporosis and osteoporotic fractures," *Epidemiologic Reviews* 7:178–208 (1985); J. Chalmers, et al., "Geographical variations in senile osteoporosis," *Journal of Bone and Joint Surgery* 52–B:667–75 (1970); G. Lewinnek, et al., "The significance and a comparative epidemiology of hip fractures," *Clinical Orthopaedics and Related Research* 152:35–43 (1980); A. Walker, "The human requirements for calcium: Should low intakes be supplemented?", *American Journal of Clinical Nutrition* 25:518–30 (1972); C. Paterson, "Calcium requirements in man: A critical review," *Postgraduate Medical Journal* 54:244–48 (1978); G. Kolata, "How important is dietary calcium in preventing osteoporosis?", *Science* 233:519–20 (1986); J. Kanis, et al., "Calcium supplementation of the diet: Not justified by present evidence," *BMJ* 298:137–40, 205–08 (1989). See generally E. Brown, *With the Grain, op. cit.*

25. R. Walker, et al., "Calcium retention in the adult human male as affected by protein intake," *Journal of Nutrition* 102:1297–1302 (1972); M. Hegsted, et al., "Urinary calcium and calcium balance in young men as affected by level of protein and phosphorus intake," *ibid.* 111:553–62 (1981). See E. Brown, *op. cit.*

26. R. Peat, *Nutrition for Women* (Eugene, Oregon: Kenogen, 1981), p. 23.

27. O. Mickelsen, "Michigan Seventh-Day Adventists: What are the benefits of a vegetarian diet?", in J. Anderson, ed., *Nutrition and Vegetarianism: Proceedings of Public Health Nutrition Update* (Health Sciences Consortium: Chapel Hill, 1981), pp. 115–17.

28. M. Shangold, "Exercise in the menopausal woman," *Obstetrics and Gynecology* 75:53S–58S (1990).

29. G. Phillips, "Hyperestrogenemia, diet, and disorders of Western societies," *American Journal of Medicine* 78(3):363–66 (1985).

30. See, e.g., A. Keys, et al., "The diet and all causes death rate in the Seven Countries Study," *Lancet* 2:58–61 (1981). See generally E. Brown, *With the Grain, op. cit.*

31. K. Khaw, E. Barrett-Connor, "Dietary potassium and stroke-associated mortality," *New England Journal of Medicine* 316(5):235–40 (1987).

32. L. Nicholson, "Focus on fiber," *Center Post* 10(9):1 (1989).

33. "Psyllium and cholesterol," *Harvard Medical School Health Letter* 13(8):1 (1988), citing *Archives of Internal Medicine* (February 1988), pp. 292–96.

34. "Mystery of high-fiber diet unraveled," *Washington Post* (October 26, 1987), p. A7; S. Siwolop, "Curbing killer cholesterol," *Business Week* (October 26, 1987), pp. 122–23.

35. "Vegetable curry, anyone?", *Harvard Health Letter* 17(12):8 (October 1992), citing *British Medical Journal* (April 18, 1992), pp. 1015–19.

Chapter Fifteen. Support from Nutritional Supplements

1. Quoted in K. Schmidt, "Old no more," *U.S. News & World Report* (March 8, 1993), p. 66–73.

2. R. Peat, *Nutrition for Women* (Eugene, Oregon: Kenogen, 1981), pp. 40–41, 48.

3. See, e.g., A. Hain, et al., "The control of menopausal flushes by vitamin E," *British Medical Journal* 7:9 (1943).

4. R. Peat, *op. cit.*, pp. 13–14.

5. G. Burton, et al, "Comparison of free alpha-tocopherol & alpha-tocopheryl acetate as sources of vitamin E in rats and humans," *Lipids* 23:834–40 (1988).

6. See L. Barbach, Ph.D., *The Pause* (New York: Penguin Books, 1993), p. 85; J. Balch, M.D., et al., *Prescription for Nutritional Healing* (Garden City Park, New York: Avery Publishing Group, 1990), p. 241.

7. L. Nachtigall, M.D., et al., *Estrogen* (New York: Harper Collins Publishers, 1991), p. 75; J. Balch, M.D., et al., *op. cit.*

8. D. Williams, "The forgotten hormone," *Alternatives for the Health Conscious Individual* 4(6):41–46 (1991), citing *Journal of the American College of Nutrition* 84(3):351.

9. L. McKeown, "Vitamin E may cut heart risk," *Medical Tribune* (November 26, 1992), p. 1.

10. J. Salonen, et al., "High stored iron levels are associated with excess risk of myocardial infarction in Eastern Finnish men," *Circulation* 86(3):803–11 (1992).
11. "Is too much iron a health risk?", *Pritikin Vantage Point* 3(1):1–3 (1992).
12. R. Peat, *op. cit.*, p. 16.
13. N. Fuchs, "Calcium controversy," *Townsend Letter for Doctors* (August/ September 1993), pp. 906–08; "Nutritional consequences of antacids for hyperacidity," *Nutrition & the M.D.* (November 1986), p. 1.
14. See G. Anderson, et al., "Effect of dietary phosphorus on calcium metabolism ...," *Journal of Nutrition* 102:1123–32 (1972); J. Froom, "Selections from current literature: Hormone therapy in postmenopausal women," *Family Practice* 8(3):288–92 (1991).
15. J. Lee, "Osteoporosis reversal: The role of progesterone," *International Clinical Nutrition Review* 10(3):384–91 (1990).
16. O. Epstein, et al., "Vitamin D, hydroxyapatite, and calcium gluconate in treatment of cortical bone thinning in postmenopausal women with primary biliary cirrhosis," *American Journal of Clinical Nutrition* 35:426–30 (1982); "Microcrystalline hydroxyapatite versus calcium gluconate," *Meta Update* 90(3):4 (March 1990); *Townsend Letter for Doctors* (December 1990), p. 863.
17. B. Dawson-Hughes, et al., "A controlled trial of the effect of calcium supplementation on bone density in postmenopausal women," *New England Journal of Medicine* 323:878–83 (1990).
18. N. Fuchs, *op. cit.*; R. Peat, *op. cit.*, p. 41.
19. D. Duston (AP), "Calcium seems to help women deal with PMS," *Brownsville Herald* (Texas), September 3, 1991, p. 14.
20. S. Thys-Jacobs, et al., "Calcium supplementation in premenstrual syndrome, a randomized trial," *Journal of General Internal Medicine* 4:183–89 (1989).
21. G. Abraham, "Nutritional factors in the etiology of premenstrual tension syndromes," *Journal of Reproductive Medicine* 28:446–64 (1983).
22. F. Facchinetti, et al., "Oral magnesium successfully relieves premenstrual mood changes," *Obstetrics and Gynecology* 78:177–81 (1991).
23. H. Fontana-Klaiber, et al., "Therapeutic effects of magnesium in dysmenorrhea," *Schweiz Rundsch Med Prax* 79(16):491–94 (1990).
24. Chart compiled by Stephane Turner, R.D., reprinted in J. Lee, *op. cit.*
25. A. Gaby, "Calcium and premenstrual syndrome," *Townsend Letter for Doctors* (October 1992), p. 810.
26. J. Balch, et al., *op. cit.*, p. 241.

27. See K. Keville, "A total approach to fighting PMS," *Vegetarian Times* (August 1986), pp. 40 ff.; D. Horrobin, "The role of essential fatty acids and prostaglandins in the premenstrual syndrome," *Journal of Reproductive Medicine* 28(7):465–68 (1983).
28. See M. Schmidt, *Childhood Ear Infections* (Berkeley, California: North Atlantic Books, 1990), pp. 99–100.
29. W. Martin, "The miracle of evening primrose oil," *Townsend Letter for Doctors* (November 1992), pp. 990–92.
30. *Ibid.*
31. U. Erasmus, *Fats and Oils* (Vancouver, Canada: Alive Books, 1989), p. 252.
32. *Ibid.*, pp. 252, 254.
33. W. Martin, *op. cit.*
34. M. Schmidt, *op. cit.*, p. 88.
35. M. Laserre, et al., "Effects of different dietary intakes of essential fatty acids ...," *Lipids* 20(4):233–77 (1985).
36. U. Erasmus, *op. cit.*, p. 258.
37. J. Booyens, et al., "Cancer: A simple metabolic disease," *Medical Hypotheses* 12:195–201 (1983) (doses of evening primrose oil equal to taking six capsules a day reduced human cancer cell lines by over 50%); D. Horrobin in *Reviews in Contemporary Pharmacotherapy* 1(1) 1990 (adding amounts of evening primrose oil equal to a human dosage of 50 grams a day entirely killed human cancer cell lines).

Chapter Sixteen. Saying No to Drugs

1. D. Barry, *Dave Barry Turns 40* (New York: Ballantine Books, 1990).
2. A. Kappas, et al., "Nutrition-endocrine interactions," *Proceedings of the National Academy of Sciences USA* 80:7646–49 (1983); D. Williams, "The forgotten hormone," *Alternatives for the Health Conscious Individual* 4(6):41–46 (1991).
3. E. Brown, L. Walker, *The Informed Consumer's Pharmacy* (New York: Carroll & Graf, 1990).
4. *Drug Facts and Comparisons*, 1993 edition (St. Louis: Facts and Comparisons), pp. 2549–52.
5. "Nolvadex reduces breast cancer recurrence," *U.S. Pharmacist* (April 1989), p. 12.
6. M. Beard, "Atrophic vaginitis: Can it be prevented as well as treated?", *Postgraduate Medicine* 91(6):257–60 (1992).

7. See, e.g., J. Cairns, "The treatment of diseases and the war against cancer," *Scientific American* 253(5):51 (1985); H. Vorherr, "Adjuvant chemotherapy of breast cancer: Reality, hope, hazard?", *Lancet* (December 19/26, 1981), pp. 1413–14; I. Tannock, "Treating the patient, not just the cancer," *New England Journal of Medicine* 317(24):1534–35 (1987); U. Abel, *Chemotherapy of Advanced Epithelial Cancer* (Stuttgart: Hippokrates Verlag GmbH, 1990), summarized by R. Moss in "Chemo's 'Berlin Wall' crumbles," *Cancer Chronicles* (December 1990), p. 4.

8. See R. Moss, *Cancer Therapy: The Independent Consumer's Guide to Non-Toxic Treatment and Prevention* (New York: Equinox Press, 1992); I. Lane, *Sharks Don't Get Cancer* (Garden City Park, New York: Avery Publishing Group, 1992).

9. J. Lee, M.D., "Slowing the aging process with natural progesterone," (Sebastopol: BLL Publishing, 1992).

10. "Dr. John Lee speaking on natural progesterone, 1992," audiotape (Sebastopol, California).

11. *Ibid.*

12. P. Hilts, "Dangers of some new drugs go undetected, study says," *New York Times* (May 27, 1990).

13. D. Orman, "... the agency (FDA) has gotten a little schizophrenic," *Townsend Letter for Doctors* 118:469 (May 1993).

14. W. Ray, et al., "Psychotropic drug use and the risk of hip fracture," *New England Journal of Medicine* 316:363–69 (1987).

15. See "Late-life love," *Harvard Health Letter* 18(1):1–3 (1992); E. Brown, L. Walker, *op. cit.*

16. J. Brody, "An alert for older Americans about preventable adverse reactions to many common drugs," *New York Times* (November 10, 1988), p. B20.

17. See, e.g., S. Guttmacher, et al., "Ethics and preventive medicine: The case of borderline hypertension," *Hastings Center Report* 11:12–20 (1981); J. Wikstrand, "Initial therapy for mild hypertension," *Pharmacotherapy* 6(2):64–72 (1986); N. Freundlich, et al., "Hypertension drugs: How much is hype?", *Business Week* (November 20, 1989), pp. 98–102; R. Antonicelli, et al., "The mild hypertension enigma," *Medical Hypotheses* 36:216–20 (1991); N. Kaplan, "Non-drug treatment of hypertension," *Annals of Internal Medicine* 102:359–73 (1985). See E. Brown, L. Walker, *op. cit.*

18. See, e.g., M. Frick, et al., "Helsinki Heart Study," *New England Journal*

of Medicine 317(2):1237–45 (1987); F. Oliver, et al., "A co-operative trial in the primary prevention of ischaemic heart disease using clofibrate," *British Heart Journal* 40:1069–1118 (1978); C. Blum, et al., "Current therapy for hypercholesterolemia," *JAMA* 261(24):3582–87 (1989). See E. Brown, L. Walker, *op. cit.*

19. J. Lee, *op. cit.*
20. P. Rylance, et al., "Natural progesterone and antihypertensive action," *British Medical Journal* 290:13–14 (1985).
21. H. Beinfeld, et al., *Between Heaven and Earth: A Guide to Chinese Medicine* (New York: Ballantine Books, 1991); J. Balch, M.D., et al., *Prescription for Nutritional Healing* (Garden City Park, New York: Avery Publishing Co., 1990); M. Wiener, et al., *Complete Book of Homeopathy* (Garden City Park, New York: Avery Publishing Co., 1989).

Chapter Seventeen. Longevity

1. R. Wilson, *Feminine Forever* (New York: Lippincott, 1966), pp. 21–22.
2. N. Angier, "Radical new view of role of menstruation," *New York Times* (September 21, 1993), p. C1.
3. R. Mishra, M.D., *Fundamentals of Yoga* (New York: Crown Publishers, 1987), p. 88.
4. R. Stocker, et al., "Ubiquinol-10 protects human low density lipoprotein more efficiently against lipid peroxidation than does alpha-tocopherol," *Proceedings of the National Academy of Sciences* 88:1646–50 (1991).
5. P. Kidd, et al., "Coenzyme Q10: Essential energy carrier and antioxidant" (HK Biomedical Consultants, August 1988).
6. J. Lee, "Slowing the aging process with natural progesterone" (Sebastopol, California; unpublished research paper); "Dr. John Lee speaking on natural progesterone, 1992," audiotape (Sebastopol: BLL Publishing, 1992).
7. G. Cowley, "Can hormones stop the clock?", *Newsweek* (July 16, 1990), p. 66; K. Schmidt, "Old no more," *U.S. News & World Report* (March 8, 1993), pp. 66–73.
8. N. Fabris, et al., "Arginine-containing compounds and thymic endocrine activity," *Thymus* 19(supp.1):S21–S30 (1992).
9. *Ibid.*
10. A. Barbul, et al., "Wound healing and thymotropic effects of arginine: A pituitary mechanism of action," *American Journal of Clinical Nutrition* 37:786–94 (1983).

11. S. Moncada, et al., "Biosynthesis of nitric oxide from L-arginine," *Biochemical Pharmacology* 38(11): 1709–15 (1989).

12. J. Balch, M.D., et al., *Prescription for Natural Healing* (Garden City, New York: Avery Publishing Co., 1990), pp. 28, 241; D. Pearson, S. Shaw, *Life Extension: A Practical Scientific Approach* (New York: Warner Books, 1982).

13. D. Pearson, et al., *ibid.*, p. 229.

14. *Ibid.*, p. 82.

15. C. Hackenthal, M.D., "Clinical experiences with DHEA," *Townsend Letter for Doctors* 117:323–24 (April 1993); K. Schmidt, *op. cit.*

16. R. Peat, *Nutrition for Women* (Eugene, Oregon: Kenogen, 1981), p. 39; K. Schmidt, *op. cit.* See the pioneering work of Roy Walford, M.D., e.g. in *Maximum Life Span* (New York: W. W. Norton & Co., 1983).

17. L. Cornaro, *Discourses on the Sober Life* (Mokelumne Hill, California: Health Research [undated]).

Chapter Eighteen. Stress, Sex, and Meditation

1. Swami Muktananda, *Play of Consciousness* (Ganeshpuri, India: Gurudev Siddha Peeth, 1978), p. 7.

2. R. Mishra, M.D., *Fundamentals of Yoga* (New York: Crown Publishers, 1987).

3. S. White, *Across the Unknown* (Columbus, Ohio: Ariel Press, 1939), p. 126. Other good books on meditation include *Touching Peace: Practicing the Art of Mindful Living* by Thich Nhat Hanh (Berkeley, California: Parallax Press, 1992) and *Journey of Awakening: A Meditator's Guidebook* by Ram Dass (New York: Bantam, 1990).

4. G. Guillaume, "Postmenopausal osteoporosis and Chinese medicine," *American Journal of Acupuncture* 20(2):105–11 (1992).

5. R. Peat, *Nutrition for Women* (Eugene, Oregon: Kenogen, 1981), pp. 7–8.

Index

187

Index

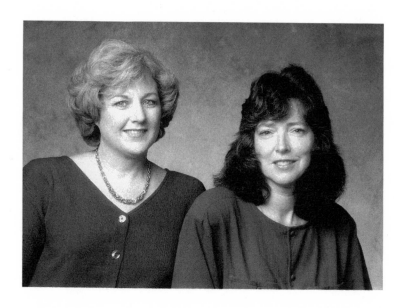

Ellen Hodgson Brown graduated from U.C. Berkeley in 1967 and from UCLA Law School in 1977, where she published her first article on the legal problems of alternative health care. She practiced law for ten years in Los Angeles before moving to Kenya and Honduras with her husband, an attorney, and children. They now live in Guatemala. Earlier books include *With the Grain: Eat More, Weigh Less, Live Longer* and *The Informed Consumer's Pharmacy* (co-authored with Lynne Walker).

Lynne Paige Walker holds a doctorate in pharmacy, a master's in Chinese herbology and acupuncture, and a doctorate in homeopathy. She worked for twelve years as a hospital pharmacist before disillusionment with the drug business and a positive experience with Oriental medicine propelled her into the work of alternative therapies. She has studied with noted holistic doctors Trevor Cook (homeopath to the Royal Family of England), Walter Strum, Bruce Waller, M.D., Jan deVries, Bernard Jensen, Francisco Eizayaga, and Robin Murphy. Dr. Walker maintains a private practice in acupuncture and homeopathy in Sun Valley, Idaho, and owns the Sun Valley Herb Company, the largest distributor of homeopathic and herbal medicines in the Pacific Northwest.

Chasteberry

? Valor II
Cistus
German Chamomaile
Acceptance — listed last
Peace & Calming II
Surrender — 3rd listing
Valor ~~III~~ 2

Coconut Oil
76° melt
Licorice ROOT
1oz/day

Black current seed oil
co Q10
Progesterone

Sun Valley
Herbs
(Idaho

Quiet Contemplative
Relaxed Wanderer
or Hsiao Yao Wan
or Xiao Yao Tang

Tongue symptoms !

DONG QUAI &
FENNEL